BRENDA DAVIS, RD, AND VESANTO MELINA, MS, RD

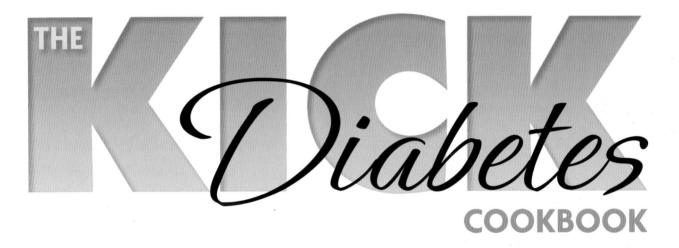

THE KICK *Diabetes* COOKBOOK

an action plan and recipes for defeating diabetes

Book Publishing Company
SUMMERTOWN, TENNESSEE

Library of Congress Cataloging-in-Publication Data

Names: Davis, Brenda, 1959- author. | Melina, Vesanto, 1942- author.
Title: The kick diabetes cookbook : an action plan and recipes for defeating
    diabetes / Brenda Davis, RD, Vesanto Melina, MS, RD.
Description: Summertown, Tennessee : Book Publishing Company, [2018]
Identifiers: LCCN 2018008177 | ISBN 9781570673597 (pbk.)
Subjects: LCSH: Diabetes—Popular works. | Diabetes—Diet therapy—Recipes. |
    Self-care, Health—Popular works. | LCGFT: Cookbooks.
Classification: LCC RC660.4 .D383 2018 | DDC 641.5/6314—dc23
LC record available at https://lccn.loc.gov/2018008177

Recipe Credits:

Adapted from *Cooking Vegan* by Vesanto Melina, MS, RD, and Joseph Forest: Zesty Black Bean Soup (p. 76), Limey Avocado Dip or Dressing (p. 105), African Chickpea Stew (p. 132), Stuffed Winter Squash (p. 140)

Adapted from *The Raw Food Revolution Diet* by Cherie Soria, Brenda Davis, RD, and Vesanto Melina, MS, RD: Garden Blend Soup (p. 73)

Adapted from *Becoming Raw* by Brenda Davis, RD, and Vesanto Melina, MS, RD: Kale Salad with Orange-Ginger Dressing (p. 88)

Adapted from drfuhrman.com/recipes/1556/fudgy-black-bean-brownies, Black Bean Brownies (p. 166)

Disclaimer: The information in this book is presented for educational purposes only. It isn't intended to be a substitute for the medical advice of a physician, dietitian, or other health-care professional.

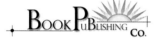

We chose to print this title on sustainably harvested paper stock certified by the Forest Stewardship Council, an independent auditor of responsible forestry practices. For more information, visit https://us.fsc.org.

Cover and interior design: John Wincek
Food styling and photography: Alan Roettinger
Stock photography: 123 RF

Printed in Canada

Book Publishing Company
PO Box 99
Summertown, TN 38483
888-260-8458
bookpubco.com

ISBN: 978-1-57067-359-7

23 22 21 20 19 18   1 2 3 4 5 6 7 8 9

CONTENTS

ACKNOWLEDGMENTS

Writing books has been likened to birthing babies. Book Publishing Company has served as a highly skilled and deeply cherished midwife, helping to birth our ten books over a span of more than twenty years. Each and every experience has been enriching, enlightening, and joyful.

It is an honor to work with our exceptionally talented editors and advisors, Cynthia Holzapfel and Jo Stepaniak. They are consistently thoughtful, articulate, and incredibly insightful. We were wonderfully privileged to have Barb Bloomfield expand and fine-tune the recipes. She has such proficiency in the kitchen and does it all with a gracious heart. We are indebted to the entire Book Publishing team, particularly Bob Holzapfel, Anna Pope, and Michael Thomas, for their expertise, energy, and encouragement. Special thanks to Alan Roettinger for his beautiful food photography.

We will be forever grateful to our dear friend Margie Colclough, who spent many months assisting us with this manuscript. She gathered an outstanding team of recipe testers and led the charge to ensure the recipes were tasty, foolproof, and easy to follow. Thank you for your incredible attention to detail and your wisdom and generosity.

We extend our heartfelt appreciation to our dedicated recipe testers: Lynn Isted, Sheanne Mosuluk, Cec Frey-McLean, Rachael Harrison, and Robin Bajer. We are deeply grateful for all the care and attention you gave to testing the recipes and for your invaluable feedback. Many thanks as well to Art Isted, Dan Mosuluk, and Bill Frey-McLean, who served as brilliant food critics.

Many thanks to *Weimar Institute's NEWSTART Lifestyle Cookbook* for inspiring the Hearty Split Pea, Lentil, and Barley Soup (p. 77), and to Chris Kalinich for contributing the recipe for Sweet Potato and Chickpea Salad (page 101), Living Light Culinary Arts Institute for contributing the recipe for Tahini-Zucchini Dip (page 115), and Sadia Badiei, RD, for contributing the recipe for Lime Bliss Balls (page 165).

Finally, we would like to thank our dear spouses, Cam Doré and Paul Davis, and our families, who have never failed to provide support, encouragement, and love throughout the process.

INTRODUCTION

Kicking Diabetes

If you receive a diagnosis of type 2 diabetes, you may wonder, Why me? Although genes may be partly to blame, diet and lifestyle bear the brunt of the burden. Your genes act as a loaded gun; however, diet and lifestyle are what typically pull the trigger. Overindulgence and underactivity, which are pervasive in our modern culture, have generated the current raging epidemics of overweight, obesity, and type 2 diabetes.

We're hardwired by nature to be attracted to the tastes of fat, sugar, and salt. When foods are eaten as they grow naturally—unprocessed and whole—they contain relatively low concentrations of these flavors. However, when fat, sugar, and salt are concentrated and used as principal ingredients in processed foods, our innate ability to control our appetites becomes unhinged.

This is no mere coincidence. Essentially, these flavors provide such pleasure that they trigger cravings and are physically addictive. Foods that are hyperconcentrated in sugar, fat, and salt stimulate the same pleasure centers in the brain that heroin, nicotine, and alcohol do. To further challenge our senses, portion sizes keep expanding. According to the Centers for Disease Control and Prevention, the average restaurant meal is four times larger than it was in the 1950s. Not surprisingly, evidence confirms that as portion sizes increase, people eat more. For anyone trying to make a living selling food, addictive flavors and larger portions mean return customers and rising sales.

To add insult to injury, the amount of physical activity we get today has dwindled dramatically since the 1950s. Every possible convenience has been developed to help reduce energy expenditure. Even if people wanted to increase their physical activity, many neighborhoods lack sidewalks and safe places for exercise. In such an environment, it's a wonder how anyone is able to maintain a healthy body weight.

In the United States, being overweight or obese is the new normal, with over 70 percent of the adult population being affected. Furthermore, many people don't know that diabetes and prediabetes are also rapidly becoming the norm, affecting an estimated half of the adult population. The good news is that by carefully controlling your diet and lifestyle, you can change the expression of your genes and dramatically diminish your risk of diabetes and other chronic diseases.

Most individuals believe that diabetes is a progressive, irreversible disease. They're taught this as a matter of fact by their health-care providers, and this viewpoint is pervasive in diabetes education resources. It follows then that conventional therapy is designed to *improve* blood glucose control—not to cure the disease. To make matters worse, some of the treatments that are most effective in controlling blood sugar (insulin injections and some oral medications) contribute to weight gain and inadvertently foster insulin resistance and disease progression. Other medications commonly used in people with diabetes can boost appetite, slow metabolism, cause fluid retention, and reduce energy (and, as a result, physical activity). In addition, conventional diabetes diets are designed to stabilize blood glucose levels, not to fight the primary drivers of the disease, insulin resistance or diminished beta cell function. So it's entirely understandable that reversal is not on the radar of most medical practitioners. Nonetheless, there's strong and consistent evidence that people who are highly motivated to reverse type 2 diabetes can succeed. A case in point is our friend Carlos, who began his healing journey over six years ago. Today he is free of the chronic diseases that nearly took his life, and his son is cancer-free as well. You can read his story below. By carefully following the guidelines in this book, you too will give yourself the best chance to reclaim your health and, like Carlos, kick diabetes for good.

CARLOS'S STORY

I was diagnosed with type 2 diabetes when I was fifty. For the next twenty years, I was injecting between 35 and 40 units of insulin (both L and N) per day. I was also on other diabetic medications, including Dia-

Beta and metformin. In total, I was taking seventeen pills a day. I had coronary artery disease and had already had one heart attack. I also had high blood pressure, early signs of kidney failure, peripheral artery disease, and chronic gout, among other ailments. I believed that my conditions were irreversible and progressive. With respect to my diabetes in particular, based on what my doctors told me and on the widely distributed literature about diabetes, I "knew" that diabetes was an irreversible disease. Then, my oldest son was diagnosed with cancer, and he decided to adopt a whole-foods, plant-based diet. To support him, my wife and I changed our diets as well.

I was being treated at UC San Francisco, so I was confident that I needed the medication I was taking and that my conditions could be managed to some extent but not reversed. What happened after I changed my diet was unbelievable to me. Within weeks I had cut my medication significantly, lost weight, and started feeling a fundamental change in my body. Today, after about a year and a half on a whole-foods, plant-based diet, I'm taking zero insulin and zero pills. My fasting glucose is now between 80 and 87 on a daily basis and my A1C is normal. My average blood pressure is now 115/70. (Even with all the medication, my blood pressure was high and never reached an average normal range.) My arteries have opened up, and I needed no procedures or surgeries. The scar tissue resulting from my heart attack has shrunk, indicating potential tissue regeneration. My kidney function is now perfectly normal, and I'm no longer taking the medication I had been prescribed for this problem. I averted (and possibly reversed) peripheral artery disease. In short, I reversed all the conditions that I "knew" were progressive and irreversible. Today I had to go to the DMV to renew my driver's license. I could not believe that I answered no to the question "do you have diabetes?" I am no longer diabetic. This all may sound incredible, but it's true. My story is supported by medical exams and records that reflect my conditions before and after I changed my diet.

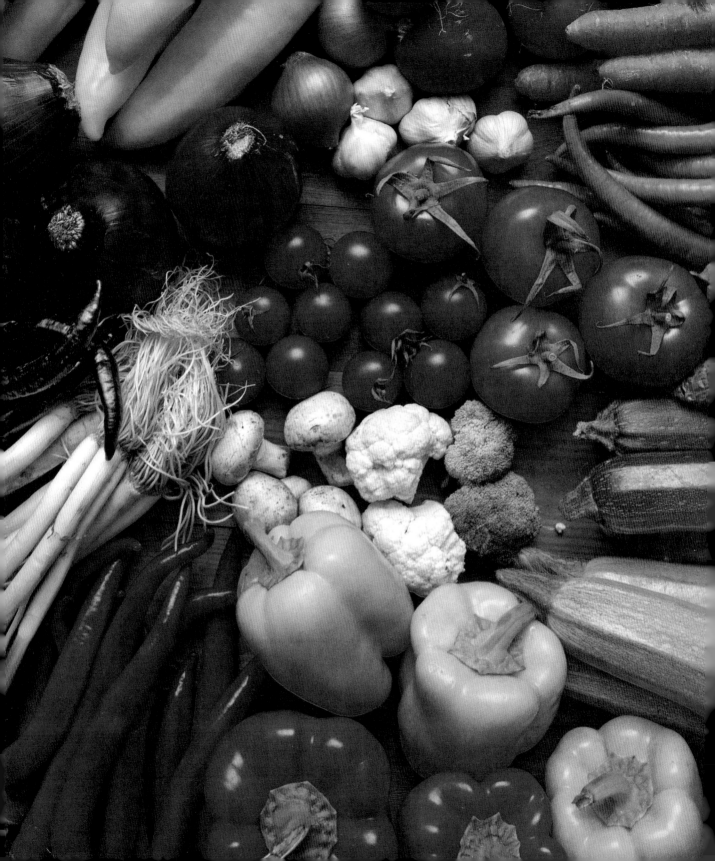

The Power and Promise of a Plant-Based Diet

1

Research has clearly demonstrated that healthy lifestyle choices could prevent 90 percent of type 2 diabetes, and there's strong consensus that diet is the kingpin. Adopting smart diet and lifestyle choices after the onset of diabetes can change the course of the disease and, in many cases, reverse it altogether.

We know this from studies of people with diabetes who made significant changes to their diets. In studies using very-low-calorie diets, reversal of insulin resistance has been reported within seven days. A more gradual reversal of insulin resistance has been reported with the use of whole-foods, plant-based diets that are less restrictive. The reason this approach is successful is because such diets disable the drivers of insulin resistance.

Plant Foods: The Key to Success

Plant foods are the primary sources of the nutrients known to protect against diabetes. Fiber (the indigestible part of plants) helps control blood sugar, lowers blood cholesterol, keeps the gastrointestinal system healthy, promotes a health-supportive mix of gut bacteria, and aids with weight loss by staving off hunger. Fiber is only found in plant foods, not in animal products. Phytochemicals, also found only in plants, improve fasting blood glucose and insulin sensitivity and reduce inflammation.

Plant foods are high in prebiotics, the component in food that nourishes the beneficial gut bacteria that reduce chronic inflammation, improve insulin sensitivity, and control blood sugar. Fermented plant foods, such as tempeh, miso, naturally pickled vegetables, and nondairy yogurts, provide friendly bacteria that aid in the maintenance of a healthy microbiome. Plant foods also contain large amounts of antioxidants and phytochemicals, compounds that help us fight the onset and progression of disease. See page 14 for a list of some of the most concentrated sources.

Highly processed foods and animal products are the primary sources of compounds that have been linked to increased insulin resistance, inflammation, gastrointestinal disorders, hormonal imbalances, high blood cholesterol levels, and hypertension. Refined carbohydrates (carbohydrate-rich foods that have been stripped of fiber and nutrients by food-processing techniques) promote overeating, inflammation, and insulin resistance. Trans fats (found mainly in partially hydrogenated oils, which are currently being eliminated from the food supply) and saturated fats (found most frequently in animal-based foods) increase insulin resistance and cholesterol levels. Other dietary factors that can increase inflammation and the harmful effects of diabetes are environmental contaminants, excessive sodium, certain food additives, and high-temperature cooking (such as grilling or frying foods).

Diet and Lifestyle: Your Focus for Defeating Diabetes

Changes in diet and other aspects of lifestyle are fundamental to restoring health. Where diet is concerned, you need to focus on disabling the drivers of insulin resistance. All of these drivers influence weight gain in some way. Even a little excess weight impairs insulin sensitivity in people with type 2 diabetes, so aim for a loss of one to two pounds (0.5–1 kg) a week. The following Kick Diabetes strategies will show you how:

Bulk up on fiber.

Include legumes, whole grains, and generous servings of vegetables and fruits throughout the day.

To reverse diabetes, aim to get at least 45–60 grams of fiber a day, depending on your body size (larger individuals will benefit by aiming for at least 60 grams per day). This translates to a minimum of 15–20 grams per meal. Particularly helpful are foods rich in soluble fiber, such as barley, beans, flaxseeds, oats, and some fruits and vegetables (apricots, asparagus, Brussels sprouts, citrus fruits, mangoes, parsnips, passion fruit, sweet potatoes, and turnips), as soluble fiber helps to stabilize blood glucose and reduce blood cholesterol levels.

TABLE 1 Fiber in common foods

FOOD (SERVING SIZE)	FIBER (G)
Beans, lentils, and split peas, cooked, 1 cup/250 ml	14–17
Avocado, 1 medium	13
Edamame or lima beans, 1 cup /250 ml	10
Peas, 1 cup/250 ml	8
Intact whole grains (barley, bulgur, Kamut berries, or spelt berries), cooked, 1 cup/250 ml	6–8
Baked potato or sweet potato, with skin, 1 medium	5–8
Flaxseeds, whole, 2 tbsp/30 ml	7
Blackberries, raspberries, 1 cup/250 ml	6–7
Vegetables, higher fiber (e.g., asparagus, broccoli, Brussels sprouts, cooked greens, green beans, okra, parsnips, squash), 1 cup/250 ml	4–6
Fruits, higher fiber (e.g., apples, blueberries, guava, kiwi, pears), 1 cup/250 ml	4–6
Oatmeal, 1 cup/250 ml	4
Almonds or sunflower seeds, ¼ cup/60 ml	4
Pasta, whole wheat, 1 cup/250 ml	4
Brown rice, cooked, 1 cup/250 ml	3.5
Peanuts, ¼ cup/60 ml	3
Vegetables, lower fiber (e.g., cabbage, carrots, cauliflower, celery, peppers, raw greens, turnips, 1 cup/250 ml	1–3.9
Fruits, lower fiber (e.g., banana, cherries, grapes, mango, melon, orange, pineapple, strawberries), 1 cup/250 ml	1–3.9
Dried fruits, ¼ cup/60 ml	2–3
Other nuts, ¼ cup/60 ml	1–2

Reduce the glycemic load (GL) of your diet.

Fill most of your plate with legumes, nonstarchy vegetables, and fruits, plus nuts and seeds (in smaller amounts). Include moderate portions of other healthy foods, such as whole grains and starchy vegetables.

The glycemic load (GL) is a rating system that estimates the impact a serving of food will have on your blood sugar. GL is related to the well-known glycemic index (GI) of foods; however, GL is even more helpful for our purposes because it includes the actual amount of carbohydrate in a standard serving. Some foods, such as watermelon, have a high GI but a low GL because the total amount of carbohydrate in a standard serving is low.

You can find extensive GI and GL indexes online. Table 2 provides a general idea of the GI and GL of some common foods. Use the following color key to help you quickly select the best options.

Foods with a low GL have a relatively small impact on blood glucose. Bear in mind that GI and GL are just one set of factors by which we judge the healthfulness of food. Some unhealthy foods, such as potato chips, have a low GI and moderate GL, while some extremely healthy foods, such as sweet potatoes, have a high GI and GL. Note that preparation can affect GI and GL, so don't be surprised if you see slightly different numbers in various tables.

You can take simple steps to reduce the glycemic impact of your meals and how much your blood sugar spikes after a meal. Among the most powerful tools is the addition of vinegar, lemon, or lime, ideally near the beginning of your meal on a salad. Even two to three teaspoons (10–15 ml) is often enough to have an effect. Cinnamon (see page 39) can reduce blood sugar spikes, as it appears to slow stomach emptying, so sprinkle it on breakfast cereal or sliced fruit.

GI (Glycemic Index)	GL (Glycemic Load)
Green = low GI (55 or less)	Green = low GL (10 or less)
Yellow = medium GI (56–69)	Yellow = medium GL (11–19)
Red = high GI (70 or more)	Red = high GL (20 or more)

TABLE 2 GI and GL of common foods

FOOD	GI	SERVING SIZE	GL
GRAINS			
Barley, cooked	28	5 oz/1 cup (150 g)	12
Bulgur wheat, boiled	48	5 oz/⅞ cup (150 g)	13
Cornflakes	81	1 oz/1 cup (30 g)	20
Millet, cooked	71	5 oz/⅞ cup (150 g)	26
Oatmeal (instant), cooked	79	1 cup (250 g)	21
Porridge from rolled oats, cooked	55	1 cup (250 g)	13
Puffed rice cakes	82	0.9 oz/ 3 cakes (25 g)	17
Quinoa, cooked	53	5 oz/⅞ cup (150 g)	13
Rice, brown, cooked	50–87	5 oz/¾ cup (150 g)	16–33
Rice, white, cooked	43–109	5 oz/¾ cup (150 g)	15–46
Rye crispbread	64	0.9 oz/2 wafers (25 g)	10
Shredded wheat	67	1 oz/1 large biscuit (30 g)	13
German pumpernickel	46	1 oz/1 slice (30 g)	6
White bread	75	1 oz/1 slice (30 g)	11
White spaghetti, cooked	49	6 oz/1½ cups (180 g)	24
Whole wheat bread	74	1 oz/1 slice (30 g)	9
Whole wheat spaghetti, cooked	44	6 oz/1½ cups (180 g)	18
LEGUMES			
Beans, lentils, dried peas, cooked	22–29	5 oz/¾ cup (150 g)	2–6
Chickpeas, cooked	31	5 oz/¾ cup (150 g)	9
Hummus	6	1 oz/2 tbsp (30 g)	0
Soybeans, cooked	18	5 oz/¾ cup (150 g)	1
NUTS			
Cashews	22	1.7 oz/⅓ cup (50 g)	3
Peanuts	14	1.7 oz/⅓ cup (50 g)	1
VEGETABLES, STARCHY			
Beets, boiled	64	2.7 oz/½ cup (80 g)	4
Carrots, boiled	39	5 oz/1 cup (150 g)	2

FOOD	GI	SERVING SIZE	GL
Corn, boiled	57	5 oz/1 cup (150 g)	13
Peas, frozen, boiled	39	2.7 oz/1 cup (80 g)	3
Potatoes, baked, russet	76	5 oz/1 small (150 g)	23
Potatoes, boiled	82	5 oz/1 small (150 g)	21
Sweet potatoes, boiled	70	5 oz/¾ cup (150 g)	22
FRUITS			
Apple, raw	36	4 oz/1 small or 1 cup chopped (120 g)	5
Banana, raw	48	4 oz/1 medium (120 g)	11
Dates	42	2 oz/7–8 small dates (60 g)	18
Grapes	46	4 oz/¾ cup (120 g)	8
Mango	41	4 oz/ ¾ cup (120 g)	8
Oranges	45	4 oz/1 small (120 g)	5
Peaches	28	4 oz/1 small (120 g)	4
Pears	38	4 oz/¾ cup (120 g)	4
Pineapple	51	4 oz/¾ cup (120 g)	8
Plums	24	4 oz/2 medium (120 g)	3
Strawberries	40	4 oz/¾ cup (120 g)	1
Watermelon	72	4 oz/¾ cup (120 g)	4
MILKS, DAIRY AND NONDAIRY			
Cow's milk, full fat	31	1 cup (250 ml)	4
Rice milk	86	1 cup (250 ml)	23
Soy beverage	15–43	1 cup (250 ml)	1–7
SNACK FOODS			
Chocolate, dark	23	1.7 oz (50 g)	6
Chocolate, milk	37	1 cup (250 ml)	9
Popcorn	72	0.7 oz/2½ cups (20 g)	8
Potato chips	54	1.7 oz/40 chips (50 g)	11
Pretzels	84	1 oz/6 pretzel twists (30 g)	17

Rethink carbohydrates.

Get your carbohydrates from whole plant foods; avoid refined carbohydrates.

Despite its shortcomings and fallacies, the trendy pro-paleo, anti-carbohydrate movement is bang-on about refined carbohydrates, such as sugar and white flour, being strongly associated with adverse health outcomes and diabetes risk. The vast majority of the carbohydrates North Americans consume fall into this category. Yet when carbohydrates come from whole plant foods, they're consistently associated with positive health outcomes. In fact the healthiest populations in the world have carbohydrate intakes ranging from 50 to 80 percent of calories! Carbohydrates are not the enemy; refined carbohydrates are. Carbohydrate-rich whole plant foods are loaded with phytochemicals, antioxidants, fiber, and other protective components, so it's a colossal mistake to lump them in with refined carbohydrates.

Forgo artificial sweeteners.

These wolves in sheep's clothing are best completely avoided.

Artificial sweeteners are not allies in the battle against diabetes. Scientific evidence suggests they don't help to cut calories, aid weight loss, or improve blood sugar control. Instead, artificial sweeteners may negatively impact blood glucose control, desensitize your taste buds to sweetness, adversely affect the growth of helpful gut bacteria, and increase hunger and sugar cravings because your body expects calories to come with sweet flavors.

If you're struggling without a low-calorie or noncaloric sweetener during your transition to a whole-foods, plant-based diet, the safest options are monk fruit sweetener and stevia. Use them in the tiniest amounts you can, and eventually eliminate them altogether.

Support a healthy gut flora.

Eat foods rich in pre- and probiotics. Avoid foods that foster an overgrowth of bad bacteria (dysbiosis).

To help overcome dysbiosis and establish health-supporting gut bacteria, boost the amount and types of fiber in your diet (see page 3). For variety, avoid using the same foods day after day. For example, instead of brown rice, try barley, Kamut berries, rye berries, or quinoa.

Eat foods rich in probiotics (see sources on page 45). Take a probiotic supplement that contains several different strains of microorganisms and opt for high dosages (at least 10–20 billion CFU per day for adults). Check the expiration date and store the supplements in the refrigerator. Also include rich dietary sources of prebiotics, such as asparagus, bananas, beans, whole grains, onions, and garlic.

Eat foods with plenty of polyphenols. These can increase the population of good bacteria in the gut and reduce some particularly nasty microorganisms. Great sources of polyphenols include almonds, blueberries, broccoli, cocoa, grapes, green tea, and onions. Minimize foods such as alcohol, artificial sweeteners, fried foods, meat, refined sugars, and white-flour products that foster the growth of bad gut bacteria.

Emphasize whole plant foods with a low caloric density.

These are foods that take up a lot of space on your plate (and in your stomach) but pack few calories per bite.

Fill up on nonstarchy fresh vegetables, fruits, and legumes. Include moderate amounts of calorie-dense foods, such as starchy vegetables and whole grains, at each meal to keep you satisfied. The amounts will depend on your weight-loss or maintenance goals. High-fat plant foods, such as avocados, nuts, and seeds, have an even higher caloric density, so keep portions of these foods small. The most calorie-dense foods of all are concentrated fats and oils, which are best avoided. In summary:

- Reduce portion sizes, except for nonstarchy vegetables, fruits, and legumes. (Starchy vegetables are listed on pages 5–6; all others are nonstarchy.)
- Avoid added fats and deep-fried foods.
- Abstain from concentrated sweeteners, such as sugar, honey, and syrups.
- Eliminate all beverages with added sugars.
- Steer clear of refined starchy foods, such as breads, white rice and pasta, muffins, crackers, cookies, and pretzels.
- Minimize snacking.

Pick plant-based protein sources.

Feature legumes (beans, peas, and lentils) at nearly every meal.

Plant protein decreases diabetes risk, while animal protein (especially processed and red meats) increases risk. Legumes are rich sources of antioxidants, fiber, and phytochemicals, whereas meats have few to none of these healthful components. In addition, red and processed meats are high in substances associated with inflammation and oxidative stress, such as carnitine (which forms trimethylamine N-oxide, known as TMAO), chemical contaminants, heme iron, N-glycolylneuraminic acid (Neu5Gc), and saturated fat.

Avoid added fats, and keep total fat intake moderate.

Get your fat mainly from whole plant foods. Focus your menu on legumes, whole grains, vegetables, and whole fruits, with a few servings of higher-fat plant foods, such as nuts, seeds, or avocado.

If you eat a variety of legumes, whole grains, vegetables, and fruits, your calories from fat will hover around 10 percent. (See table 3 for more precise amounts.) Each serving of high-fat, whole plant foods (nuts, seeds, or avocado) will add 3–5 percent to this number, depending on your total caloric intake. One serving equals two tablespoons (30 ml) of nuts or seeds, one tablespoon (15 ml) of nut butter, or one-quarter of a medium avocado. So, adding one high-fat food would increase calories from fat to 13–15 percent, two would be 16–20 percent, three 19–25 percent, and four 22–30 percent. So for most people trying to lose weight, adding no more than two to four servings is a reasonable target, depending on your body size and weight-loss goals.

Avoid any use of oil and other concentrated fats. These foods provide about 120 calories per tablespoon (15 ml) and have the lowest nutrient density (the fewest nutrients per calorie) of all foods. When fighting diabetes, especially if you're overweight, you want every calorie that crosses your lips to be bursting with protective components.

Include reliable sources of essential fatty acids.

Flaxseeds, chia seeds, hemp seeds, and walnuts are particularly good sources.

Some fats are labeled "essential" because we can't make them—they must come from our food. There are two essential fatty acids: linoleic acid (an

TABLE 3 Calories from fat in a variety of foods

FOOD	% CALORIES FROM FAT
VEGETABLES	
Most vegetables	0–10
Basil, bok choy, cauliflower, cilantro, corn, kale, lettuce (most varieties), parsley, spinach, baby zucchini	11–19
Avocados	69–79
Olives	89
FRUITS	
Most fruits	0–11
Durian	30
Coconut	83
LEGUMES	
Most beans, lentils, split peas	3–4
Chickpeas	14
Soybeans	43
Peanuts	72
GRAINS	
Barley, buckwheat, Kamut berries, spelt berries, wheat berries, wild rice	3–6
Brown rice, cornmeal, millet	7–13
Oats, quinoa	14–16
NUTS AND SEEDS	
Chia seeds, flaxseeds, hemp seeds	50–69
Almonds, cashews, pistachios, poppy seeds, pumpkin seeds, sesame seeds, sunflower seeds	70–79
Brazil nuts, hazelnuts, pecans, pine nuts, walnuts	80–89

FOOD	% CALORIES FROM FAT
ANIMAL PRODUCTS	
Beef, ground, 80% lean, broiled	60
Cheese, Cheddar	72
Milk, full fat	52
Salmon, cooked with dry heat	37

omega-6 fatty acid) and alpha-linolenic acid (an omega-3 fatty acid). Omega-6 fatty acids are found in poppy, pumpkin, sesame, and sunflower seeds, as well as in whole grains and many other plant-based foods. Omega-3 fatty acids are plentiful in chia seeds, flaxseeds, hemp seeds, and walnuts.

In general we don't have to worry much about getting enough omega-6s; getting enough omega-3s is more of an issue. A day's supply of omega-3s can be obtained from 1 tablespoon (15 ml) of ground flaxseeds, 1 ounce (30 g) of walnuts, 1½ tablespoons (22 ml) of chia seeds, or 3 tablespoons (45 ml) of hemp seeds. People with diabetes have a more difficult time converting omega-3s from plant foods, so fish, (a direct source of the larger, more active long-chain omega-3 fatty acids, EPA and DHA) is often touted as a superfood for these individuals. While fish is more healthful than meat, it's one of the most concentrated sources of environmental contaminants.

Safer sources of long-chain omega-3s are microalgae—the tiny plants in the sea that are the actual source of EPA and DHA consumed by fish! You can find omega-3 supplements that have been extracted from cultured microalgae. If you take 200–300 mg EPA and DHA daily, or even just two or three times a week, you would get an amount of omega-3s similar to what you would get from fish—without the contaminants.

Reduce your sodium intake to no more than 1,500 mg per day.

The easiest way to do that is to build your diet around whole plant foods and prepare your meals from scratch.

Processed foods often contain a hefty dose of salt to add flavor. The amount of salt in some processed foods may surprise you; ounce for ounce, cornflakes have more salt than salted peanuts! (See table 4, page 12.)

TABLE 4 Sodium content of common foods*

FOOD	SODIUM CONTENT (MG)
Salt, 1 tsp (5 ml)	2,300
Pepperoni pizza, 12-inch diameter (30 cm)	5,959
Canned beans, 1 cup (250 ml)	750–950
Soup, 1 cup (250 ml)	600–900
Macaroni and cheese, boxed, 1 cup (250 ml)	869
Pickle, dill, 1 medium	833
Miso, 1 tbsp (15 ml)	634
Tomato sauce, ½ cup (125 ml)	450
Cottage cheese, ½ cup (125 ml)	410
Canned corn, drained, 1 cup (250 ml)	336
Pretzels, 1 oz (30 g)	352
Soy sauce or tamari, 1 tsp (5 ml)	300–350
Canned beans, low sodium, 1 cup (250 ml)	250–350
Canned tuna, 3 oz (90 g)	301
Olives, 10 small	270
French fries, medium (5 oz/150 g)	290–890
Canned tomatoes, ½ cup (125 ml)	225
Cornflakes, 1 oz (30 g)	204
Ketchup, 1 tbsp (15 ml)	178
Cheese, Colby, 1 oz (30 g)	169
Bread, whole wheat, 1 slice	150
Potato chips, 1 oz (30 g)	148
Crackers, Ritz, 5	141
Peanuts, dry-roasted, salted, 1 oz (30 g)	116

Source: USDA Nutrient Database.

*Compare to the recommended maximum daily sodium intake of 1,500 mg.

To keep your sodium intake low, rely on whole foods as the foundation of your diet and prepare foods yourself instead of using packaged, jarred, or canned items. If you use any processed foods, look for products labeled as "low salt" or "reduced-sodium," and keep your intake moderate. Use salt-free herb blends for cooking, and select seasonings that don't list salt among the ingredients. Omit salt or use a smaller amount of salt than a recipe calls for.

Use fresh or frozen vegetables and dried beans instead of canned when possible. If using jarred or canned foods, rinse them well to remove some of the sodium or look for salt-free brands. Limit the use of pickled products—they're soaked in salt!

Go lightly on added salt while cooking and at the table or omit it completely. Ask restaurant chefs to do the same. When cooking at home, add any salt near the end of the cooking time; you can use less that way. We register a salty taste when salt is on the surface of a food (such as a salted cracker) because that immediately contacts our taste buds. Use lemon or lime juice on foods instead of salt.

Maximize your intake of phytochemicals and antioxidants.

Fill your plate with a wide variety of colorful plant foods daily.

Choosing whole plant foods (especially organic) that cover the full spectrum of the rainbow is the key to a diet rich in phytochemicals and antioxidants. Cooking reduces these protective compounds. In general, the higher the heat and the longer the cooking time, the greater the loss. On the other hand, sprouting and fermenting significantly increase the phytochemical content. The absorption of phytochemicals from raw foods can also be increased by breaking down the foods, as with blending, chopping, grating, processing, pureeing, or chewing the foods well.

Drinking vegetable juice can be a practical way to boost antioxidant and phytochemical intake. If you have diabetes and drink vegetable juices, limit your intake to between four and eight ounces (120–250 ml) per day. Vegetable juices are best when they're freshly pressed. To keep calories down, don't include fruits and use only small amounts of beets or carrots. A great combination is leafy greens, celery, cucumber, ginger, turmeric root, and lemon or lime.

30 ANTIOXIDANT- AND PHYTOCHEMICAL-RICH SUPERSTARS

- Almonds
- Apples
- Beans (especially black/red)
- Berries (especially black/blue)
- Cherries
- Cilantro
- Cinnamon
- Citrus fruits
- Cruciferous vegetables (such as broccoli and broccoli sprouts)
- Cocoa powder
- Cranberries
- Dill
- Fennel
- Garlic
- Green tea
- Greens, dark leafy
- Ginger
- Grapes (red or black)
- Lentils
- Onions
- Peanuts
- Plums (purple)
- Pomegranates
- Saffron
- Sesame seeds and tahini
- Soybeans
- Sunflower seeds
- Tomatoes
- Turmeric
- Walnuts

Minimize your intake of chemical contaminants.

Eat plants; choose organic options for foods that are typically highly contaminated.

Chemical contaminants can disrupt the functioning of our cells and damage the liver and pancreas. If you can't afford to buy everything organic, select organic for products that potentially have the highest pesticide levels. Primarily, foods that are eaten with the skin (such as apples, berries, peaches, and pears) pose a greater risk than those eaten with the peel removed (such as bananas, kiwi, melons, and pineapples). Eat more raw foods. Washing doesn't completely remove pesticides, but washing and peeling produce will reduce pesticide content. You can obtain a more complete list of pesticides in foods from the Environmental Working Group website (ewg.org/foodnews). Print out their list to take with you when you go shopping or download it to your phone.

Moderate your intake of rice and rice products and avoid hijiki seaweed, as these can be significant sources of arsenic. Select whole foods rather than highly processed foods or deep-fried foods. Use wet cooking methods, such as braising, steaming, and stewing, rather than barbecuing, broiling, and frying. If you use high temperatures for cooking, don't blacken or overcook foods. Avoid oils in cooking, but if you do use oils, never allow them to smoke.

Finally, use stable materials, such as glass, for storing and reheating food in the microwave, instead of plastic. Steer clear of imported canned foods because they may have lead seams, and avoid foods stored in lead-glazed ceramic or leaded glassware. Look for canned goods with BPA-free linings.

Meet the RDA for all nutrients.

In particular, get the Recommended Dietary Allowance of chromium, magnesium, potassium, the antioxidants, and vitamins B_{12} and D.

Many people with diabetes need more of certain vitamins and minerals, especially chromium, magnesium, and potassium; the antioxidant vitamins A (as carotenoids), C, and E; and vitamins B_{12} and D, in order to ensure nutritional adequacy, restore insulin sensitivity, and promote healing. Eating plant-based foods, plus taking a few supplements, will ensure that you get these nutrients. To be sure you get enough, here are simple steps you can take:

Antioxidant vitamins. The antioxidant vitamins C and E and carotenoids are abundant in plants, so the move to a whole-foods, plant-based diet usually provides sufficient amounts. Vegetables and fruits are rich in carotenoids and vitamin C. Vitamin E is most concentrated in higher-fat plant foods (such as almonds, avocados, hazelnuts, peanuts, pine nuts, sunflower seeds, and wheat germ) and in broccoli, butternut squash, dark leafy greens, kiwi, and red peppers.

Vitamin B_{12}. Having insufficient vitamin B_{12} can cause problems with fasting blood glucose, oxidative stress, and inflammation in individuals with diabetes. People who are taking metformin are also at increased risk of being low in vitamin B_{12}, as metformin reduces B_{12} absorption. In addition, everyone over fifty, whether they eat a plant-based diet or not, is at risk for being low in vitamin B_{12} because our ability to absorb it can decrease as we age. Whole plant foods are not reliable sources of vitamin B_{12}; the real source is bacteria. To ensure adequate intakes, see the guidelines on page 23.

Vitamin D. A growing number of people in the United States get less vitamin D than they need: over 40 percent of adults overall, over 80 percent of black adults, and almost 70 percent of Hispanic adults. There's mounting evidence that a lack of vitamin D can increase the risk for developing diabetes and increase the seriousness of existing conditions.

While it's possible to produce enough vitamin D by safely exposing your skin to the sun, the intensity of the sun at your latitude, the amount of cloud cover, the amount and type of clothing you wear, your age, and whether you're carrying excess body fat all can affect vitamin D production. It's challenging to get enough vitamin D from food; see the guidelines on page 24.

Chromium. Chromium enhances the action of insulin and plays an important role in the metabolism of carbohydrates, fat, and protein. Broccoli is a chromium superstar with about 22 mcg per cup (250 ml). Other rich plant sources of this nutrient are Brazil nuts, green beans, lentils, pears, potatoes, prunes, strawberries, tofu, tomatoes, and whole grains (especially barley and oats). Whether people with diabetes would benefit from taking chromium is uncertain; many medications interact with chromium, so be sure to check with your physician if you are considering a chromium supplement.

Magnesium. Magnesium helps control blood sugar by regulating insulin secretion from the pancreas. People with diabetes are more likely to be low in magnesium because high blood sugar causes magnesium to be excreted in the urine. The richest sources are dark chocolate, nuts (such as almonds, Brazil nuts, cashews, pine nuts) and seeds (such as chia, flax, poppy, pumpkin, sesame, and sunflower). Other good sources are avocado, corn, daikon radishes, dark green leafy vegetables, legumes (including soyfoods), pea shoots, and whole grains (such as Kamut, quinoa, spelt, and wheat sprouts).

Potassium. Potassium stimulates insulin production. If you're on blood pressure medication, your potassium levels may fall, so your health-care provider may tell you to increase your intake of potassium-rich foods. However, if you have kidney disease due to your diabetes, your health-care provider may tell you to restrict potassium-rich foods, although this recommendation is controversial.

In general, people with diabetes should maximize potassium intake. Bananas are often touted as the best source, but many foods outrank them, including acorn squash, bamboo shoots, black turtle beans, black-eyed peas, Chinese cabbage, green soybeans, kiwi, lima beans, potatoes, sweet potatoes, tomato sauce, and taro.

Ensure adequate hydration.

Drink about eight glasses of water a day.

People with diabetes are at a higher risk for dehydration because high blood sugar levels deplete fluids. Dehydration can cause skin to become dry, itch, and crack, increasing the risk of infection. Water is the ideal hydrator—it doesn't raise blood sugar, and it has zero calories. A good target goal is to drink six to eight glasses a day for women and eight to ten glasses a day for men. If plain water doesn't do it for you, try adding a few slices of citrus fruit or cucumber, a sprig of mint or lemon balm, or some frozen berries to either still or carbonated water. Other good options are teas (especially green teas, but also herbal, black, or white tea); vegetable juices made with celery, cucumber, leafy greens, ginger, lemon, or

TABLE 5 Top diabetes food friends and foes

TOP DIABETES FOOD FRIENDS	TOP DIABETES FOOD FOES
Beans, peas, and lentils	Alcohol
Berries	Beverages with added sugar
Fresh fruit	Deep-fried foods
Green leafy vegetables	Full-fat dairy products
Herbs and spices	Grilled meat or poultry
Intact whole grains (see page 35)	Processed foods with added fat, sugar, and salt
Nuts	Red and processed meats
Other vegetables	Solid fats
Seeds	Sugar, syrups, and sweets
Water	White flour and white rice products

CAN EVERYONE OVERCOME TYPE 2 DIABETES?

Type 2 diabetes can be defeated by most people but not everyone. Individuals with the best chance of reversal are those who produce enough insulin but whose insulin isn't doing its job due to insulin resistance. Individuals who can't reverse the disease are those who don't make enough insulin. It can be devastating to make the lifestyle changes that will reverse insulin resistance only to discover that your pancreas is too damaged to reverse your diabetes. In this case, you may require injected insulin for the rest of your life because your pancreas function can no longer meet your body's insulin needs.

However, you can take heart that overcoming insulin resistance itself will dramatically improve your health and quality of life. Restoring your body's insulin sensitivity will reduce your risk for many conditions, including heart disease, hypertension, certain types of cancer, and dementia. Overcoming insulin resistance also means that you'll need the lowest possible insulin doses, which will effectively reduce your risk for the most dreaded complications of diabetes.

lime; and unsweetened nut or soy milk. If you're a coffee drinker, monitor your blood sugar levels after drinking coffee; if you have a particularly negative reaction, switch to decaf or tea. If you do drink coffee, stick to black.

Steer clear of sodas, energy drinks, sports drinks, flavored water, vitamin water, fruit beverages, fruit punch, and sweetened iced tea or coffee. Alcohol can raise blood sugar levels, increase appetite, and impair judgment, as well as damage the liver and increase blood pressure and triglycerides. If you imbibe from time to time, keep your intake as low as possible and avoid making alcohol part of your daily routine.

The Kick Diabetes Lifestyle

Where lifestyle is concerned in kicking diabetes, physical activity is key, but every choice matters. Incorporate the following strategies for implementing a lifestyle that will support your dietary changes:

- **Set goals and be sure to measure your progress.** Write down your goals in life and what it's going to take to achieve them. Spell out a plan that will allow for incremental progress that's realistic. Then keep track of what you're eating, how much activity you're participating in, and what your blood glucose levels are.

- **Get a support team.** Get your family and friends on board with the changes you need to make. Work with your health-care providers and let them know about your plan.

- **Get rid of foods that aren't nutritious, and buy the foods that support health and healing.** Don't risk temptation by having foods in your house that will derail your success. Give them away. Replace them with nutritious whole foods.

- **Be prepared for challenges.** Not everyone around you may support your efforts; even your physician might be skeptical. Your friends and coworkers may encourage you to be in social settings that will sabotage your results. You could get discouraged about doing things that are new to you or be tempted to eat foods you shouldn't, especially when you're under stress. Don't let challenges stop you! Continue on, keep your goals in mind, and know that the more you improve, the better your health will be.

- **Make physical activity a part of your daily life—just like eating and sleeping.** Walk or engage in other physical activity for ten to fifteen minutes (or longer) after every meal. Once that comes easily, add thirty minutes of activity each day, and then work up to forty-five to sixty minutes of activity each day.

- **Make adequate sleep a priority in your life; an average of eight hours per night is appropriate for most people.** Practice a relaxing bedtime routine, and go to bed and get up at about the same time each day, even on weekends.

- **Identify your sources of significant stress and develop strategies to effectively manage them.** Take at least thirty minutes a day to do something you love and look forward to. Learn and practice stress-management techniques.

- **Establish and maintain strong social ties.** Studies report a 50 percent increase in the longevity of individuals with the most-active social lives. Socialize daily and spend time with good friends.

Now that you understand the basics of the Kick Diabetes diet and life-style to ensure success, you may be wondering what this all means in terms of what to eat. Chapters 2 and 3 take a closer look at the foods you need to focus on and how to incorporate them into your daily diet to achieve your ultimate goal of kicking diabetes. Then, be sure to enjoy all the delicious recipes that follow in chapter 4.

Meals and Menus to Kick Diabetes

The next steps toward kicking diabetes involve choosing the best foods, planning meals and menus, and getting practical advice to support your success. Whether you're a whiz in the kitchen or don't know where to begin, there are plenty of ways to accomplish your transition to plant-based eating.

It can take up to three to four weeks to rewire your taste buds and for your gut bacteria to adjust to the increased amount of fiber in a whole-foods, plant-based diet. A recent study reported that sugar cravings disappeared in over 85 percent of people within six days of giving up sugar and artificial sweeteners. Be prepared for sensory adjustments that take a little time. Once your taste buds become accustomed to the amazing flavors, textures, and aromas of fresh whole foods, foods that are overly fatty, sugary, and salty will seem downright disgusting.

Design Your Own Kick Diabetes Plant-Based Plate

Food guides are meant to help you design a diet that ensures all your nutrient needs are met on a daily basis. The Kick Diabetes Plant-Based Plate is intended specifically for adults with type 2 diabetes. It's rich in protective nutrients, minimizes harmful components, and meets the recommended nutrient intakes. What follows is an overview of the foods in each group and two menus that are adjusted for different activity levels.

When you're following this guide, you don't need to meet the minimum recommended servings from every food group every day. Instead, aim to have your average intakes reach those goals over time. You can arrange meals or snacks in various ways and still meet recommended intakes for all nutrients, so there's plenty of flexibility. Special guidelines are given for five nutrients—vitamin B_{12}, vitamin D, calcium, iodine, and omega-3 fatty acids—in a section on the opposite page called Essential Extras.

You'll see that certain foods that may have been regulars on your menus are missing from The Kick Diabetes Plant-Based Plate. This guide is built around whole plant foods while excluding the two categories most strongly linked to increased diabetes risk: highly processed foods and animal products.

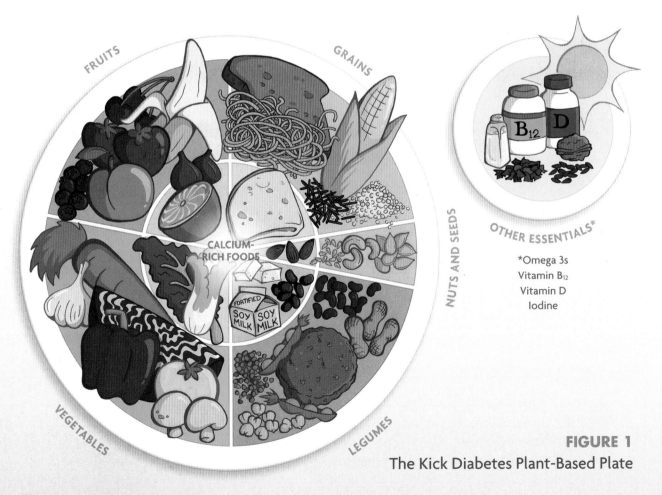

FIGURE 1
The Kick Diabetes Plant-Based Plate

TABLE 6 Kick diabetes food groups: optimal servings and serving sizes

FOOD GROUP	SERVINGS PER DAY	FOOD EXAMPLES AND SERVING SIZES	CALCIUM-RICH FOODS 5–8 SERVINGS PER DAY
Nonstarchy Vegetables	5 or more 7+ even better!	Raw or cooked vegetables, ½ cup (125 ml); raw leafy vegetables, 1 cup (250 ml); vegetable juice, ½ cup (125 ml)	Bok choy, broccoli, collard greens, kale, napa cabbage, okra, 1 cup (250 ml) cooked, or 2 cups (500 ml) raw
Fruits	3 or more	Whole fruit, medium-sized; fruit, raw or cooked, ½ cup (125 ml); dried fruit, ¼ cup (60 ml)	Oranges, 2; dried figs, ½ cup (125 ml)
Legumes	3 or more	Cooked beans, peas, or lentils, bean pasta, or tofu or tempeh, ½ cup (125 ml); raw peas or sprouted lentils, mung beans, or peas, 1 cup (250 ml); vegetarian meat substitute, 1 oz (30 g); fortified soy milk, 1 cup (250 ml)	Black or white beans, 1 cup (250 ml); calcium-set tofu, ½ cup (125 ml); fortified soy milk or soy yogurt, ½ cup (125 ml)
Whole Grains and Starchy Vegetables	2 or more	Cooked whole grains or starchy vegetables, ½ cup (125 ml); 1 oz (30 g) very dense whole-grain bread (see page 35)	—
Nuts and Seeds	2–3	2 tbsp (30 ml) nuts or seeds; 1 tbsp (15 ml) nut or seed butter	Almonds or sesame seeds, ¼ cup (60 ml); almond butter or tahini, 2 tbsp (30 ml)
Herbs and Spices	3 or more	¼–½ tsp (1–2 ml) ground spice; 1 tsp (5 ml) dried herbs; 1 tbsp (15 ml) fresh herbs	—

Essential Extras

Vitamin B$_{12}$

People age sixty-five or older or adults of any age on metformin:

- Daily: Take a supplement providing 100–1,000 mcg vitamin B$_{12}$. (Monitor your status; your physician will adjust accordingly.)

Adults under age sixty-five choose *one* of the following:

- Daily: Take a supplement providing 25–100 mcg vitamin B$_{12}$.
- Two to three times a week: Take a supplement providing 1,000 mcg vitamin B$_{12}$.
- Daily: Consume at least three servings of foods fortified with vitamin B$_{12}$ that provide at least 2 mcg vitamin B$_{12}$ per serving. The Daily Value

(DV) for vitamin B$_{12}$ used on food labels is 6 mcg, so if a food provides 33 percent of the DV, it provides 2 mcg.

Vitamin D

Get daily vitamin D from sunlight, fortified foods, a supplement, or a combination of all three:

- **Sunlight.** Expose the face and forearms to *warm* sunlight (from 10:00 a.m. to 2:00 p.m.) without sunscreen for at least fifteen minutes for light-skinned people, twenty minutes for dark-skinned people, or thirty minutes for people over the age of seventy.
- **Fortified foods or supplements.** The minimum recommended intake for vitamin D is 15 mcg (600 IUs) up to age seventy and 20 mcg (800 IUs) over age seventy. For people with diabetes, especially if they're overweight, a vitamin D supplement of 25–50 mcg (1,000–2,000) per day is advised.

Calcium

Calcium-rich foods are those in various food groups that are particularly high in this mineral. They are shown in the inner circle of The Kick Diabetes Plant-Based Plate. In table 6 (page 23), they appear in the column at the right. Become familiar with high-calcium plant foods and incorporate them into your meals regularly. Recommended intakes for calcium are as follows:

- 1,000 mg per day for women age nineteen to fifty and men age nineteen to seventy
- 1,200 mg per day for women over fifty and men over seventy
- To meet recommendations, aim for five to eight servings of high-calcium plant foods daily. (The balance will come in smaller amounts from other plant foods.) Each serving of the following foods provides approximately 150 mg of calcium:
- 2 cups (500 ml) raw bok choy, broccoli, collard greens, kale, or napa cabbage
- 1 cup (250 ml) cooked bok choy, broccoli, collard greens, kale, mustard greens, napa cabbage, or okra; black or white beans
- ½ cup (125 ml) calcium-set tofu, dried figs, fortified nondairy milk, cooked soybeans, or soy nuts

- ¼ cup (60 ml) almonds
- 2 tablespoons (30 ml) almond butter or tahini
- 2 oranges

If you fall short of the recommended number of servings of calcium-rich foods, you can top up your intake with a calcium supplement.

Iodine

You can get your day's recommended intake of 150 mcg iodine from a multivitamin-mineral supplement or from about ⅓ teaspoon (2 ml) iodized salt. Salty seasonings, such as Bragg Liquid Aminos, soy sauce, tamari, and typical Celtic, Himalayan, or sea salts are not sources of iodine. Sea vegetables, such as kelp, are rich in iodine, but amounts vary greatly and can sometimes be excessive. Check labels, although iodine levels may not always be listed.

Omega-3 Fatty Acids

Include at least *one* of the following daily; each serving provides about 2.5 g of omega-3s:

- 1 tablespoon (15 ml) ground flaxseeds
- 1½ tablespoons (22 ml) chia seeds
- 3 tablespoons (45 ml) hemp seeds or walnuts

Along with the smaller amounts of omega-3s from other plant foods, this will meet the needs of both women and men. People with diabetes may also be well advised to take a supplement of 200–300 mg microalgae-based EPA/DHA at least two to three times a week.

Fine-Tuning Your Food Step by Step

Kicking diabetes is possible, but it takes a solid commitment to lifestyle changes. It doesn't, however, require perfection. It's a process. The target servings shown on The Kick Diabetes Plant-Based Plate are your ultimate goal, but you can get there one step at a time. For each food group, we suggest three possible steps to your goal. If you need to take smaller steps, that's all right. Do what works for you. If you slip up, don't worry; that's normal. Just get back on track right away. Extend your walk an extra fifteen minutes; cut back on calories a little at your next meal. Trust the process, and trust yourself.

Nonstarchy Vegetables

KICK DIABETES TARGET: 7 or more servings per day (include a rainbow of colors)

LEVEL 1: 5 servings per day (1–2 leafy greens; 3–4 other vegetables)

LEVEL 2: 6 servings per day (2 leafy greens, 1 yellow or orange; 3 other vegetables)

LEVEL 3: 7 or more servings per day (3 or more leafy greens; 1 or more each of yellow or orange, red, purple or blue, white or beige vegetables)

BEST CHOICES

- Dark leafy greens are the most nutrient-dense of all foods, with broccoli, bok choy, collard greens, kale, mustard greens, and okra being good calcium sources. Some others are high in oxalates that reduce calcium absorption; beet greens, spinach, and Swiss chard are healthy options but not good sources of calcium.
- All other nonstarchy vegetables are great choices—eat them to your heart's content.
- Organic vegetables are preferred; minimize your exposure to potentially harmful chemicals.
- Eat a rainbow of colors to maximize the quantity and variety of protective compounds.
- The fresher, the better. Nothing beats homegrown vegetables, so if you can, frequent farmer's markets and produce stands or start gardening.

TIPS FOR SUCCESS

- *Have a giant salad as a main dish every day.* This means including a variety of delicious greens; several different-colored vegetables; protein sources, such as chickpeas, lentils, or smoked tofu; a filling addition, such as cooked cubed sweet potatoes, butternut squash, or Kamut berries; and a fat source, such as a nut- or seed-based dressing or sliced avocado. Many of the salad recipes in this book are hearty enough to serve as a main dish (see pages 84–102) .

- *For something warming, load a stew or soup with vegetables, including greens.* Use frozen vegetables if that's easier for you. Dark leafy greens, such as collards, kale, and spinach, are widely available in the supermarket frozen-foods section.

- *Have ½ cup (125 ml) of steamed dark leafy greens three times a day.* This is powerful medicine! See the recipe on page 121.

COMMON QUESTIONS

Are frozen, canned, and jarred vegetables good choices?

Fresh is generally best for maximum nutrition. However, vegetables are usually frozen soon after they've been picked, so their nutrients are well preserved. Canned vegetables lose some of their water-soluble nutrients, may be high in added sodium (unless no- or low-sodium options are chosen), and are often packed in cans with liners containing bisphenol A (BPA), a chemical found in hard plastic that's been linked to a variety of health problems. Choose BPA-free cans or glass jars.

What are the best ways to cook vegetables?

Steaming results in the greatest nutrient retention. Microwaving and blanching also minimize nutrient losses. Boiling causes greater losses of vitamins and minerals through heat and discarded water. Baking or roasting can destroy vitamins (but not minerals) and create harmful by-products (see pages 14–15). The least-desirable methods are those that use very high temperatures and concentrated oils, such as deep-frying. Although a quick sauté can preserve nutrients, it can add a lot of fat and calories if oils are liberally used. For sautéing, replace oil with vegetable broth, water, or wine.

Fruits

KICK DIABETES TARGET: 3 or more servings per day

LEVEL 1: 2 servings per day (any fresh fruit)

LEVEL 2: 3 servings per day (any fresh fruit)

LEVEL 3: 3 or more servings per day (1 of berries, 1 of citrus, 1 or more of other fruit)

BEST CHOICES

- Berries provide a lot of fiber and phytochemicals and have a low glycemic index, so they're an exceptional choice.
- Citrus fruits are high in protective phytochemicals and have less impact on blood sugar than some other fruits.
- All other fresh fruits are healthy options, although bananas and dates contain more carbohydrates and calories than most other fruits, so they have a higher glycemic load. (See "A Note about Sweeteners," page 56, for information about using dates in the recipes in this book.)
- Fresh fruits are best, but frozen fruits are also good choices. Canned or jarred fruits are acceptable if they're packed in water, although there are greater nutrient losses with canned fruits and the sugars in them are more rapidly absorbed into the bloodstream. Avoid fruits that are canned in syrup or contain added sugar.

TIPS FOR SUCCESS

- *Have fruit with your morning meal.* Have at least 2 servings (a total of 1 cup/250 ml) of fruit with breakfast.
- *Use fruit as your go-to dessert.* Fresh fruit (sliced or whole), fruit salad, fruit-based ice cream (see Tutti Frutti Ice Cream, page 161), and baked fruit make delectable treats.
- *Add fruit to salads.* Enjoy some blueberries, sliced mango, or strawberries with your salad greens.
- *Pick fruit if hunger strikes.* To make the fruit even more filling, add a little natural peanut butter, nut butter, or tahini, and top it with a sprinkle of cinnamon (see page 39).

COMMON QUESTIONS

How much fruit is too much?

It depends on what else you're eating. If you're trying to lose weight and are eating all the recommended servings of other food groups, 3 or 4 servings of fruit is a reasonable target. If you're eating fewer calories than you need, there's no set limit on whole fresh fruits.

Is the fructose in fruit a problem?

The short answer is no. The body's ability to handle fructose is seldom overwhelmed by consuming whole fruit. Fruits also are loaded with protective phytochemicals, antioxidants, vitamins, and minerals, as well as valuable fiber that slows the absorption of the sugars. In fact, the more fruit that people consume, the lower their risk of diabetes.

However, fructose itself is a potentially problematic sugar that, when consumed in excess, may result in nonalcoholic fatty liver disease. So drinks and processed foods made with sugars and syrups that are concentrated sources of fructose should be avoided.

Are dried fruits and fruit juices OK for people with diabetes?

Dried fruits are much higher in calories and have a greater impact on blood sugar than fresh fruits, so although they're healthy, they should be used sparingly. Avoid dried fruits with added sugars. Fruit juices are best avoided because they're quickly absorbed into the bloodstream and lack the fiber of whole fruits. In addition, it's easy to drink a lot of juice in a short time. You can get through one cup (250 ml) of orange or apple juice in a minute, but it would take much longer to eat two oranges or apples. Fruit water is a wonderful option. Simply add citrus slices, strawberries, or other fruit or berries to a pitcher of water and let the water steep for eight to twelve hours in the refrigerator for a refreshing, fruity-tasting, sugar-free beverage.

Legumes (beans, lentils, split peas)

KICK DIABETES TARGET: 3 or more servings per day

LEVEL 1: 2 servings per day (beans, lentils, peas, soy milk, split peas, tempeh, tofu, veggie meats)

LEVEL 2: 3 or more servings per day (at least 1 serving of whole legumes, lentils, or split peas)

LEVEL 3: 3 or more servings per day (at least 2 servings of whole legumes, lentils, or split peas)

BEST CHOICES

- Whole beans, chickpeas, split peas, and fresh peas are exceptional choices, brimming with fiber, plant protein, vitamins, minerals, and phytochemicals. Their consumption is strongly associated with diabetes risk reduction. For preparation information, see pages 53–54, as well as the many outstanding recipes in this book that contain legumes.

- Sprouted mung beans, peas, and lentils are good choices and safe to consume raw. Larger beans need to be cooked after sprouting.

- Traditional soy products are very healthful, with organic options being your best bet. Tofu and tempeh are well known as being protective against disease. Tempeh, a fermented product, is relatively high in fiber. Tofu is extremely versatile and provides readily available plant protein.

- Hummus is popular and available in many flavors and variations (see pages 113–114). Commercial varieties can be high in sodium, so always read the labels or make your own.

- Bean pasta is a rapidly rising star, with types based on a variety of legumes. The advantages over traditional pasta are extensive, especially for people with diabetes. Bean pasta provides about half the carbohydrate, double the fiber, and triple the protein of regular pasta.

TIPS FOR SUCCESS

- *Have beans for breakfast.* Many people around the world enjoy beans or lentils with their morning meals. If this strikes you as unusual, consider how tempting it would be to have a bean-based breakfast burrito, Golden Scrambled Tofu and Veggies (page 65), or Beans, Greens, and Sweet Potato with Tahini-Lime Sauce (page 64).

- *Top a Full-Meal Salad (see page 96) with plant-protein superstars.* Add chickpeas, black beans, grilled tempeh, smoked tofu, or peas.

- *Add a bean, lentil, or pea soup to your meal, along with a salad.* Many of the soup recipes in this book contain legumes and can be served as a main course.

- *Make legumes the main event.* Get creative when it comes to lunches and dinners. For centuries numerous cultures have relied on these as dietary staples. Indian, South American, Asian, and African cuisines include many delicious legume dishes.

COMMON QUESTIONS

How can I get more comfortable eating beans and lentils when they cause gas?

Beans and lentils cause gas because they contain a very healthy type of carbohydrate (oligosaccharides) that isn't broken down and digested in the small intestine. It makes its way into the large intestine and provides a feast for the bacterial inhabitants. Gas is a normal by-product of digestion. The following suggestions will help to keep gas production tolerable:

- *Reduce the oligosaccharides in beans.*
    - Use fresh instead of dried beans, as their oligosaccharide content is much lower, or select canned beans, as canning reduces oligosaccharide content. Choose unsalted canned beans or rinse them well; rinsing will further decrease the oligosaccharides.
    - Buy only as many dried beans as you can use within a few months.
    - Soak beans for six to eight hours; discard the soaking water and rinse the beans well before putting them in fresh water and cooking.
    - Sprout legumes before cooking them. Sprouting converts oligosaccharides into more-digestible sugars.
- *Start with small portions*, then gradually increase your intake. In this way, healthy gut flora will flourish and become accustomed to the dietary shift, and unhealthy flora will get crowded out.
- *Cook beans thoroughly.* When beans are undercooked, they're more difficult to digest and lead to digestive problems.
- If you're using canned beans, *rinse them well.*
- *Select small legumes*, as they are easier to digest. The least problematic are skinless, split legumes, such as mung dal (split mung beans), red lentils, and split peas. In general, these will produce less gas than large beans, such as lima or kidney beans.
- *Pick options with fewer oligosaccharides.* Choose tofu and bean products that are fermented, such as tempeh and miso.
- *Use seasonings that counteract the production of intestinal gas.* Black pepper, cinnamon, cloves, garlic, ginger, turmeric, and the Japanese seaweed kombu are all prized for their ability to diminish gas production.
- *Improve your gut flora.* Take probiotics in supplement form or use them in the preparation of fermented foods, such as vegan cheeses, yogurts, and other dishes.
- *Avoid overeating.* Eat smaller meals; stop when you are 80 percent full.
- *Avoid foods with added fructose or sugar alcohols.* The small intestine isn't equipped to handle large quantities of fructose, so undigested molecules move on to the large intestine. Similarly, sugar alcohols, such as maltitol, sorbitol, and xylitol, are not completely absorbed and are fermented by bacteria in the colon.
- *Consider a digestive enzyme supplement.* Find one that is targeted toward bean digestion.

Are canned beans OK for people with diabetes?

Canned beans are definitely OK, but they can be high in sodium and some have added sugar, so read labels. Canned baked beans typically have added sugar; it's wise to make baked beans at home so you can control the ingredients. Many companies offer no- or low-sodium products, and some provide BPA-free cans. You can reduce the sodium by about 40 percent by rinsing canned beans well before using them. For convenience, cook beans in large batches and freeze them in 1½- or 2-cup (375- or 500-ml) portions in freezer bags or jars.

Are veggie meats an acceptable option?

These are relatively processed products. However, they're high in protein and very low in carbohydrate, so they can be useful for people with insulin resistance. In some products the protein used has been extracted with toxic chemicals, such as hexane; select organic products to eliminate this concern. Many veggie meats are high in added fat and salt; check labels. Some are based on whole foods (such as burgers made with black beans and quinoa); these are great options. You can also assemble your own homemade versions.

Whole Grains and Starchy Vegetables

KICK DIABETES TARGET: 2 or more servings per day

LEVEL 1: Include 1 or no refined products. The balance should be whole grains or starchy vegetables.

LEVEL 2: Eliminate refined products. Choose 1 colorful starchy vegetable (corn, sweet potato, winter squash) and 1 or more intact whole grains.

LEVEL 3: Eliminate refined products. Choose 1 or more colorful starchy vegetables and 1 or more intact whole grains. Include other whole grains that are listed with or above rolled grains in the whole-grain hierarchy (see figure 2, page 35).

Portion control is important for this food group. Stick mainly to starchy vegetables and whole grains that have a lower glycemic index and load. Products with a high glycemic index can have an impact on blood glucose and triglycerides that is similar to that of more-refined products. Starchy vegetables (which includes breadfruit, corn, green peas, plantains, potatoes, pumpkins, sweet potatoes, taro, and winter squash) are higher in carbohydrate than nonstarchy vegetables. Although nonstarchy vegetables provide about 5 grams of carbohydrate per serving, starchy vegetables provide about triple that amount, similar to that of whole grains. Yellow and orange starchy vegetables provide two nutrients not available from whole grains: vitamin A (as carotenoids) and vitamin C. Of course, there is considerable variability within each group, with some nonstarchy vegetables (such as beets) having slightly more carbohydrate than most, and some starchy vegetables (such as butternut squash) having less carbohydrate than most.

Instead of eating foods made from whole-grain flours, become comfortable with cooking whole (intact) grains and using them in place of baked goods, bread, and packaged cereals. You'll find great information on cooking intact grains on page 56 and will be enjoying a wide variety of new flavors and textures in no time!

BEST CHOICES

- Color is a key to optimal choices. Starchy vegetables with the deepest color—orange, yellow, or purple—have the greatest antioxidant and phytochemical content. For grains, red or black quinoa and rice are higher in these protective components than beige quinoa or brown rice.

- The less processed the better. Leave the skin on starchy vegetables to increase their nutrition and fiber content. Use intact whole grains (not grains that have been shredded, flaked, or ground into flour). Many products labeled "whole grain" contain added fat, sugar, salt, flavors, colors, and preservatives; read labels carefully. The whole-grain hierarchy on page 35 is a good guide. Eat as high up on the hierarchy as possible.

- Include a variety of grains, as each one has its own strengths. Among the true grains, Kamut, oats, spelt, and wheat are the richest in protein. Barley has the lowest glycemic index, and oats have the highest soluble fiber content. The pseudograins, quinoa and buckwheat, are more concentrated in protein and trace minerals than many true grains. Each starchy vegetable has its unique advantages. Sweet potatoes are highest in carotenoids and trace minerals; winter squash provides more folate.

TIPS FOR SUCCESS

- *Include a starchy vegetable or intact whole grain at each meal.* This will make meals more satisfying and help to avoid the temptation to eat between meals.

- *Have an intact whole grain (such as brown rice or millet) or steel-cut oats at breakfast.*
- *Add whole grains or starchy vegetables to soups and salads.* For lunch, sprinkle intact whole grains or cooked sweet potato cubes on your salad. Add butternut squash or barley to soup.
- *Serve stuffed baked potatoes for dinner.* Stuffed sweet potatoes offer a nutritional advantage, but regular baked potatoes are fine too, especially when they're topped or filled with high-fiber beans. And be sure to eat the skin! Serve steamed dark leafy greens or a salad on the side.
- *Enjoy a vegetable curry or stir-fry over black rice, red quinoa, or another intact whole grain.*

COMMON QUESTIONS

Are whole grains healthy foods?

Absolutely! Grains provide about half the world's protein and fiber. Whole grains are rich in B vitamins (especially thiamin and niacin) and vitamin E. They're good sources of copper, iron, manganese, magnesium, phosphorus, selenium, and zinc, plus a variety of phytochemicals and antioxidants.

Are grains essential for a healthy diet?

No. There are no nutrients in grains that can't be derived from other foods. One approach is to eat your daily quota of vegetables, fruits, legumes, nuts, and seeds, and then vary your grain intake based on your energy (caloric) needs. If your energy needs are very low, your allowance for grains will be low. If you're moderately or very active, you can afford to eat more grains.

Should everyone avoid gluten?

No. While the 1 percent of the population with celiac disease must be vigilant about avoiding gluten, and another estimated 6–10 percent may suffer from non-celiac gluten sensitivity, most people can tolerate gluten. Vary the grains you eat, and include several gluten-free grains, such as brown rice, buckwheat, millet, and quinoa, in your rotation.

Are starches for thickening sauces off-limits because they're refined?

No. While these are highly refined, generally only a small amount is required per serving. If you use 2 tablespoons (30 ml) of arrowroot starch, cornstarch,

FIGURE 2 Kick Diabetes Whole Grain Hierarchy

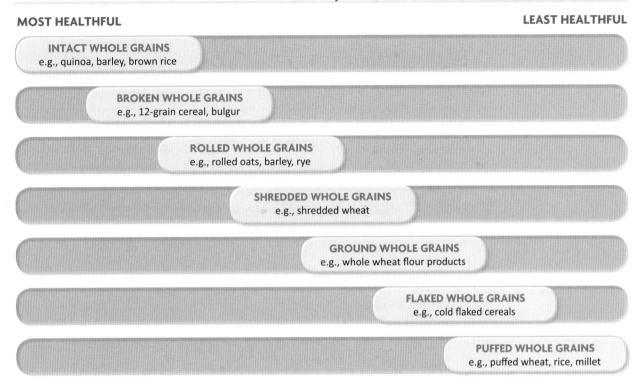

MOST HEALTHFUL   **LEAST HEALTHFUL**

INTACT WHOLE GRAINS
e.g., quinoa, barley, brown rice

BROKEN WHOLE GRAINS
e.g., 12-grain cereal, bulgur

ROLLED WHOLE GRAINS
e.g., rolled oats, barley, rye

SHREDDED WHOLE GRAINS
e.g., shredded wheat

GROUND WHOLE GRAINS
e.g., whole wheat flour products

FLAKED WHOLE GRAINS
e.g., cold flaked cereals

PUFFED WHOLE GRAINS
e.g., puffed wheat, rice, millet

or potato starch to thicken a sauce, it typically amounts to about ¾ teaspoon (4 ml) per person.

Are foods derived from grains (oat bran, wheat bran, wheat germ) healthy choices?

Although oat bran, wheat bran, and wheat germ aren't technically whole grains, they do have nutritional benefits. Oat bran can provide viscous fiber, which helps to control blood sugar. Wheat bran can be useful for people who suffer from constipation; however, caution is warranted because it can reduce mineral absorption. Wheat germ can add vitamin E to granola or muesli. In general, eating the whole grain is the best option.

Is it OK to include bread?

Yes, but very selectively. Because bread is often yeasted to make it light and fluffy, the carbohydrate in bread is rapidly absorbed and has a big impact on blood sugar. Bread can also be high in sodium and lower in fiber than intact whole grains. But some breads are more healthful than others. Sprouted breads (made from sprouted grains rather than flour, and dehydrated or baked at a low temperature) are reasonable choices. Breads made from sprouted-grain flours are less desirable than breads made from whole sprouted grains.

Usually the denser the bread, the more slowly the nutrients are absorbed and the more healthful it is. Very heavy breads (those that you can practically stand on!) are best, such as German pumpernickel. Light, fluffy whole wheat bread might have a GI of 74, while heavy German pumpernickel has a GI of about 48. The bottom line is that most of the grains you eat should be intact whole grains. If you include bread, pick wisely and have it infrequently, not daily.

Nuts and Seeds

KICK DIABETES TARGET: 2–3 servings per day

LEVEL 1: 1–2 servings per day, including ½ or 1 serving of an omega-3-rich choice (chia seeds, ground flaxseeds, hemp seeds, or walnuts)

LEVEL 2: 2–3 servings per day, including 1 serving of an omega-3-rich choice

LEVEL 3: 2–3 servings per day, including 1 serving of an omega-3-rich choice plus 1 serving of a vitamin E–rich choice (almonds, hazelnuts, peanuts, sunflower seeds)

NOTE: In this guide we include peanuts and peanut butter in the nuts and seeds group. Although peanuts are botanically legumes, they're used like nuts for culinary and nutritional purposes.

BEST CHOICES

- *Variety is the key*, as the nutrition contribution of nuts and seeds is quite diverse. Almonds and sunflower seeds are the vitamin E superstars. Almonds and chia, poppy, and sesame seeds are rich in calcium. Most seeds, pine nuts, and cashews are rich in iron and zinc. Brazil nuts are selenium superstars, and chia and pumpkin seeds are richest in magnesium. Walnuts and pecans appear to be champions in terms of antioxidant content. Peanuts are particularly high in protein.

- *Include at least one omega-3 choice: walnuts or chia, flax, or hemp seeds.* The absorption of omega-3 fatty acids is improved by grinding chia seeds and flaxseeds.

- *Be sure seeds are part of the mix.* Seeds are higher in protein and fiber and more concentrated in essential fatty acids (both omega-6 and omega-3 fatty acids) than nuts (except for walnuts).

- *When possible, choose nuts and seeds that are raw, soaked, sprouted, and dehydrated.* Soaking and sprouting increase the content and availability of nutrients, phytochemicals, and antioxidants. Roasting at temperatures above 248 degrees F (120 degrees C) can cause the formation of dangerous chemicals, but soaking and sprouting do not.

TIPS FOR SUCCESS

- *Add omega-3-rich seeds or walnuts to a breakfast bowl (see page 59).* You'll need about 1 tablespoon (15 ml) of ground flaxseeds, 1½ tablespoons (22 ml) of chia seeds, or 3 tablespoons (45 ml) of hemp seeds or walnuts to fulfill your omega-3 requirement.

- *Add 1–2 tablespoons (15–30 ml) nuts or seeds to salads.* Almonds, pumpkin seeds, and sunflower seeds are excellent choices.

- *Use seeds, nuts, or their butters as your salad-dressing base.* These are the perfect nutrient-rich replacements for oils in dressings (see the recipes on pages 104–109).

- *Use nuts or seeds in main dishes.* Add walnuts or sunflower seeds to patties or loaves, add pine nuts or hazelnuts to pilafs, or throw a few peanuts or cashews into a stir-fry.

- *Enjoy a few unshelled nuts for a snack or dessert.* Crack open two or three walnuts or five or six other nuts and serve them with sliced fresh fruit for a simple but satisfying snack or dessert.

- *Use nuts or seeds to top fruit salad, fruit-based ice cream (see Tutti Frutti Ice Cream, page 161), or baked fruit.* Sprinkle nuts or seeds on fruit desserts for added flavor and nutrient absorption and to slow the absorption of fruit sugar.

COMMON QUESTIONS
Aren't nuts and seeds high in fat and calories?

Yes, about 75–85 percent of the calories in nuts and 55–75 percent of the calories in seeds are from fat. They provide 500–800 calories per cup (250 ml)! So although they're valuable foods, they should be eaten in small amounts, not by the bowlful.

Are nuts and seeds OK for people with diabetes?

Absolutely! In fact they're more than OK—they're important. Among all the plant-based foods, nuts have the least impact on blood sugar. In addition, they deliver essential nutrients, fiber, phytochemicals, and antioxidants.

Is coconut a healthy choice?

Yes, it's acceptable, but only in small amounts, primarily as a flavor booster. Unlike true nuts, which feature monounsaturated fats, and seeds, which have mostly polyunsaturated fats, coconut contains mostly saturated fat. To enhance the flavor of foods without adding much fat, sprinkle 1 tablespoon (15 ml) of unsweetened shredded dried coconut over a breakfast bowl (see page 59) or fruit dessert. If a recipe calls for coconut milk (which has about 450 calories per 1 cup/250 ml), replace it with thick unsweetened soy or cashew milk, and add 1 teaspoon (5 ml) of coconut extract per 1 cup (250 ml) of nondairy milk.

Herbs and Spices

KICK DIABETES TARGET: 3 or more servings per day

Herbs and spices are of tremendous value in a diabetes-reversal diet because of the wealth of protective phytochemicals and antioxidants they contain.

LEVEL 1: 1 or more servings per day

LEVEL 2: 2 or more servings per day

LEVEL 3: 3 or more servings per day

BEST CHOICES

- Cinnamon seems to show the most promise for slowing blood glucose absorption or stabilizing blood sugar, although cayenne, cloves, curry powder, fenugreek, garlic, ginger, marjoram, rosemary, and sage may also be of value.
- Turmeric is the anti-inflammation superstar. Basil, black pepper, cardamom, cinnamon, cloves, garlic, ginger, fennel, nutmeg, and rosemary all have inflammation-quenching abilities.

- For the greatest antioxidant action, cloves lead the pack. Allspice, basil, bay leaves, chiles, cinnamon, curry powder, ginger, lemon balm, marjoram, mint, dry mustard, oregano, paprika, saffron, sage, thyme, and turmeric are in the running too.

TIPS FOR SUCCESS

- *Spice up breakfast.* Allspice, cinnamon, cloves, ginger, and nutmeg combine well with sweet breakfasts. Basil, cayenne, garlic, oregano, rosemary, thyme, and turmeric are great additions to savory breakfasts.
- *Infuse hot teas with herbs or spices.* Use cinnamon, cloves, fennel, ginger, lemon balm, mint, or turmeric.
- *Add fresh herbs to salads.* Basil, chives, cilantro, dill, mint, parsley, oregano, and thyme are wonderful herbs for salads.
- *Add herbs and spices to salad dressings.* Basil, cayenne, garlic, ginger, mustard, and turmeric all add a welcome jolt of flavor. Mustard also acts as an emulsifier.
- *Season soups, stews, and other dishes with plenty of herbs and spices.*

COMMON QUESTIONS

Does it matter if herbs are fresh or dried?

Both are excellent choices. For a salad or as a garnish, fresh is best. If you're cooking herbs for fifteen minutes or longer, either fresh or dried will do. Whole dried spices will keep for three to four years, ground spices for two to three years, dried herbs for one to three years, and seasoning blends for one to two years. Store dried herbs and spices in a cool, dry spot, away from heat.

Are some types of cinnamon potentially toxic?

Yes. The cinnamon that's commonly used throughout North America is called cassia cinnamon and contains a compound called coumarin, which is toxic to the liver, especially in large amounts. Some countries have suggested upper intake limits of no more than ⅓–1 teaspoon (2–5 ml) daily for a 176-pound (80-kg) person. Either limit your intake of cassia cinnamon or use Ceylon cinnamon instead. Although less widely available (it can be purchased online) and more expensive, Ceylon cinnamon contains very little coumarin. The taste is milder but pleasant. Although most studies on cinnamon and blood sugar reduction were done using cassia cinnamon, there is evidence that Ceylon cinnamon provides similar advantages.

Getting Ready for Your Culinary Adventure

Transitioning to plant-based eating may seem a little overwhelming at first, so think of it as a culinary adventure with delightful surprises. There are a number of things you can do to make your plant-based journey go a little smoother:

- *Gather the essential kitchen equipment.* This means having a good chef's knife, paring knife, cutting board, mixing bowls, measuring spoons and cups, saucepans, baking pans, and baking sheets. Consider investing in a heavy-duty, high-powered blender and a food processor. These will help you prepare dressings, frozen-fruit ice creams (see Tutti Frutti Ice Cream, page 161), spreads, and sauces in a jiffy. A multipurpose programmable pressure cooker makes cooking beans a breeze. For more ideas, see the comprehensive list on page 49.

- *Take a plant-based cooking class.* Make it a priority to explore what's available locally or online. A cooking school specializing in plant-based whole foods will familiarize you with ingredients, recipes, and flavor combinations to help you find healthy replacements for your favorite comfort foods and broaden your culinary horizons.

- *Find resources that keep your creative juices flowing.* Cookbooks, magazines, websites, and videos can inspire and motivate you to try new things. Embrace the adventure.

- *Surround yourself with like-minded people who eat plant-based diets.* One fundamental requirement for success is finding people who will support you in your transition. Look for plant-based groups, meetups, and events in your area. If local sources are few and far between, find support online.

Kick Diabetes Menus

The following two menus are designed to provide powerful results for people with type 2 diabetes. Each menu can supply 1,600, 2,000, or 2,400 calories (kcal), depending on the serving sizes consumed. The first menu features fast and easy preparation; the second requires moderate preparation time. Typically, the 1,600-calorie menus are suitable for weight loss in women. The 2,000-calorie menus are suitable for weight loss in men and weight maintenance in women. The 2,400-calorie menus are suitable for weight maintenance in men. Adjust the calorie content of these menus to suit your needs.

MENU 1 Fast and easy preparation

MEAL	FOOD	SERVING SIZE		
		1,600 CALORIES	2,000 CALORIES	2,400 CALORIES
Breakfast	Simple Morning Muesli (page 58) with blueberries, peaches	1 cup (250 ml)	2 cups (500 ml)	2 cups (500 ml)
	Unsweetened fortified nondairy milk	1 cup (250 ml)	1 cup (250 ml)	1 cup (250 ml)
	Lemon-ginger tea or tea of choice	As desired	As desired	As desired
Lunch	Five-Day Salad (page 85)	2 cups (500 ml) or more	2 cups (500 ml) or more	2 cups (500 ml) or more
	Carrot, grated	1	1	1
	Smoked tofu	½ cup (125 ml/120 g)	½ cup (125 ml/120 g)	½ cup (125 ml/120 g)
	Hummus and Lime Dressing (page 106)	¼ cup (60 ml)	¼ cup (60 ml)	¼ cup (60 ml)
	Pumpkin seeds	—	1 tablespoon (15 ml)	¼ cup (60 ml)
Afternoon Snacks (or Lunch or Dessert)	Fresh orange	1	1	1 or 2 fruits of choice
	Strawberry-infused water	As desired	As desired	As desired
Dinner	Curry in a Hurry Soup (page 78)	2 cups (500 ml)	2 cups (500 ml)	2½ cups (750 ml)
	Brown or black rice	½ cup (125 ml)	½ cup (125 ml)	1 cup (125 ml)
	Cashews	2 tablespoons (30 ml)	2 tablespoons (30 ml)	3 tablespoons (45 ml)
Snacks or Desserts	Tutti Frutti Ice Cream (page 161)	¾ cup (185 ml)	¾ cup (185 ml)	1 cup (250 ml)
	Unsweetened fortified nondairy milk	½ cup (125 ml)	1 cup (250 ml)	1 cup (250 ml)
	Apple or fruit of choice	1	1	1
	Walnuts	2 tablespoons (30 ml)	—	—

Number of servings from each food group

FOOD GROUP	RECOMMENDATION	1,600 CALORIES	2,000 CALORIES	2,400 CALORIES
Legumes	3 or more	3	3½	3½
Nonstarchy Vegetables	5 or more	5	5	5
Starchy Vegetables and Grains	2–6	2	3	3
Fruits	3 or more	5	5½	7
Calcium-Rich Foods	5–8	4½	5½	5½
Nuts and Seeds	2–3	2	2+	3
Herbs and Spices	3 or more	3+	3+	3+

If you're not losing weight as expected (1–2 pounds/0.5–1 kg per week), you'll need to exercise more, if possible, and slightly reduce your caloric intake. Analyses are done using unsweetened fortified soy milk, which is higher in protein than other nondairy milks. However, other unsweetened fortified nondairy milks could be used instead, as the menus provide more than enough protein for most people. The menus are designed to meet recommended nutrient intakes as long as vitamins B_{12}, D, and iodine requirements are met (see pages 182–183). If you use a multivitamin mineral supplement, choose one that includes calcium, iodine, and vitamins B_{12}, D, and E. Menus 1 (page 41) and 2 (page 43) feature the "good" carbs, mainly from whole grains and legumes, as well as good fats that provide beneficial omega-3 fatty acids. They also contain abundant plant protein and provide all the essential amino acids. The small amount of vitamin B_{12} comes from the fortified nondairy milk.

The nutrients provided by each menu can be compared to the recommendations for your age and gender as shown on pages 182–183.

Nutritional analysis for 1,600-calorie menu: calories: 1,626, protein: 73 g, fat: 48 g, carbohydrate: 252 g, dietary fiber: 44 g, calcium: 1,111 mg, iron: 22 mg, magnesium: 407 mg, phosphorus: 1,400 mg, potassium: 3,471 mg, sodium: 1,248 mg, zinc: 8.3 mg, thiamin: 1.3 mg, riboflavin: 1.5 mg, niacin equivalents: 15 mg, vitamin B_6: 1.6 mg, folate: 442 mcg, vitamin B_{12}: 1.2 mcg, vitamin A: 871 mcg RAE, vitamin C: 205 mg, vitamin E: 5 mg, vitamin K: 275 mcg, omega-6 fatty acids: 12 g, omega-3 fatty acids: 3.2 g

Percentage of calories from: protein 18%, fat 23%, carbohydrate 59%

Nutritional analysis for 2,000-calorie menu: calories: 2,008, protein: 91 g, fat: 57 g, carbohydrate: 310 g, dietary fiber: 54 g, calcium: 1,492 mg, iron: 26 mg, magnesium: 605 mg, phosphorus: 1,966 mg, potassium: 4,243 mg, sodium: 1,416 mg, zinc: 10 mg, thiamin: 1.6 mg, riboflavin: 2.1 mg, niacin equivalents: 18 mg, vitamin B_6: 1.7 mg, folate: 475 mcg, vitamin B_{12}: 1.8 mg, vitamin A: 879 mcg RAE, vitamin C: 212 mg, vitamin E: 6 mg, omega-6 fatty acids: 14.2 g, omega-3 fatty acids: 4.5 g

Percentage of calories from: protein 17%, fat 24%, carbohydrate 59%

Nutritional analysis for 2,400-calorie menu: calories: 2,413, protein: 104 g, fat: 81 g, carbohydrate: 351 g, dietary fiber: 61 g, calcium: 1,561 mg, iron: 30 mg, magnesium: 856 mg, phosphorus: 2432 mg, potassium: 4,784 mg, sodium: 1,420 mg, zinc: 12 mg, thiamin: 1.8 mg, riboflavin: 2.1 mg, niacin equivalents: 23 mg, vitamin B_6: 2.1 mg, vitamin B_{12}: 1.8 mg, folate: 512 mcg, vitamin A: 880 mcg RAE, vitamin C: 226 mg, vitamin E: 6 mg, omega-6 fatty acids: 23 g, omega-3 fatty acids: 6 g

Percentage of calories from: protein 16%, fat 28%, carbohydrate 56%

MENU 2 Moderate preparation

MEAL	FOOD	SERVING SIZE		
		1,600 CALORIES	**2,000 CALORIES**	**2,400 CALORIES**
Breakfast	Beans, Greens, and Sweet Potato with Tahini-Lime Sauce (page 64)	½ recipe	½ recipe	½ recipe
	Peach, mango, or Fresh Fruit Salad (page 159)	1 cup (250 ml)	1 cup (250 ml)	1 cup (250 ml)
	Green tea or tea of choice	As desired	As desired	As desired
Lunch	The Big Easy Bowl (page 131) or Full-Meal Salad (page 96)	The Big Easy Bowl (page 131) with ½ cup (125 ml) each grains and beans; 1 tbsp (15 ml) chia seeds	The Big Easy Bowl (page 131) with ½ cup (125 ml) grains, 1 cup (250 ml) beans, 1 tbsp (15 ml) chia seeds	The Big Easy Bowl (page 131) with 1 cup (250 ml) each grains and beans; 3 tbsp (45 ml) chia seeds
	Creamy Hemp Dressing (page 107)	2 tbsp (30 ml)	¼ cup (60 ml)	¼ cup (60 ml)
	Mint-infused water	As desired	As desired	As desired

MEAL	FOOD	SERVING SIZE		
Dinner	African Chickpea Stew (page 132)	1½ cups (375 ml)	2 cups (500 ml)	2 cups (500 ml)
	Kale Salad with Orange-Ginger Dressing (page 88)	⅞ cup (220 ml)	1 cup (250 ml)	1½ cups (375 ml)
Snacks or Desserts	Raw Vegetable Platter (page 91)	2 cups (500 ml) raw veggies	2 cups (500 ml) raw veggies	2 cups (500 ml) raw veggies
	Heartwarming Hummus (page 113)	—	3 tbsp (45 ml)	¼ cup (60 ml)
	Berries	1 cup (250 ml) berries	1 cup (250 ml) berries	1 cup (250 ml) berries
	Unsweetened fortified nondairy milk	1 cup (250 ml) soy milk	1 cup (250 ml) soy milk	1 cup (250 ml) soy milk

Number of servings from each food group

FOOD GROUP	RECOMMENDATION	1,600 CALORIES	2,000 CALORIES	2,400 CALORIES
Legumes	3 or more	3½	4½	4½
Nonstarchy Vegetables	5 or more	11	12	13
Starchy Vegetables and Grains	2–6	3½	4	4½
Fruits	3 or more	4	4	4½
Calcium-Rich Foods	5–8	5–6	6	8
Nuts and Seeds	2–3	2	2½	2½
Herbs and Spices	3 or more	4+	4+	5+

Nutritional analysis for 1,600-calorie menu: calories: 1,614, protein: 67 g, fat: 52 g, carbohydrate: 244 g, dietary fiber: 59 g, calcium: 1,004 mg, iron: 20 mg, magnesium: 664 mg, phosphorus: 1,709 mg, potassium: 4,723 mg, sodium: 1,234 mg, zinc: 12 mg, thiamin: 2.3 mg, riboflavin: 1.6 mg, niacin equivalents: 28 mg, vitamin B_6: 2.5 mg, folate: 934 mcg, vitamin B_{12}: 1 mcg, pantothenic acid: 5 mg, vitamin A: 3,052 mcg RAE, vitamin C: 336 mg, vitamin E: 12 mg, omega-6 fatty acids: 20 g, omega-3 fatty acids: 4 g

Percentage of calories from: protein 16%, fat 27%, carbohydrate 57%

Nutritional analysis for 2,000-calorie menu: calories: 2,035, protein: 86 g, fat: 65 g, carbohydrate: 306 g, dietary fiber: 74 g, calcium: 1,167 mg, iron: 25 mg, magnesium: 891 mg, phosphorus: 2,195 mg, potassium: 5,833 mg, sodium: 1,562 mg, zinc: 15 mg, thiamin: 2.8 mg, riboflavin: 1.9 mg, niacin equivalents: 34 mg, vitamin B_6: 3 mg, folate: 1,283 mcg, vitamin B_{12}: 1 mcg, pantothenic acid: 5.5 mg, vitamin A: 3,367 mcg RAE, vitamin C: 413 mg, vitamin E: 13 mg, omega-6 fatty acids: 25 g, omega-3 fatty acids: 5 g

Percentage of calories from: protein 16%, fat 27%, carbohydrate 57%

Nutritional analysis for 2,400-calorie menu: calories: 2,414, protein: 99 g, fat: 79 g, carbohydrate: 360 g, dietary fiber: 90 g, calcium: 1,439 mg, iron: 30 mg, magnesium: 1,048 mg, phosphorus: 2,644 mg, potassium: 6,466 mg, sodium: 1,735 mg, zinc: 19 mg, thiamin: 3.3 mg, riboflavin: 2.1 mg, niacin equivalents: 40 mg, vitamin B_6: 3.6 mg, folate: 1,410 mcg, vitamin B_{12}: 1 mcg, pantothenic acid: 6 mg, vitamin A: 3,578 mcg RAE, vitamin C: 476 mg, vitamin E: 15 mg, omega-6 fatty acids: 30 g, omega-3 fatty acids: 9 g

Percentage of calories from: protein 16%, fat 28%, carbohydrate 56%

Meal Timing and Frequency

Regular mealtimes are important because they help stabilize blood sugar, control appetite, and achieve weight loss. When people put time and thought into planning what they're going to eat and when, their meals tend to be more balanced. When there isn't any advance preparation, people have a greater tendency to overeat and to eat too quickly. Also be aware that insulin and diabetes medications can cause hypoglycemia.

Try to eat your first meal within one and a half hours of getting up in the morning. Other meals can be eaten about every four to six hours after that. Legumes (beans, peas, and lentils) can be good allies for maintaining your blood glucose level between meals. If you aren't taking diabetes medications or insulin, how often you eat and when you eat are matters of personal preference, as long as you eat healthy foods in reasonable quantities. The important thing is what works for *you*. Some people love a hearty breakfast, but others have a limited appetite after waking and a light breakfast works best for them. What seems to be most important is maintaining consistency from day to day.

Regardless of meal timing, learning to recognize and respect hunger is vital to weight management. Avoid overeating or depriving yourself when you're famished. If you think you're hungry, drink a glass of water, then wait fifteen minutes to ensure that you're not mistaking thirst for hunger. If you're really hungry, have a piece of fruit with 2 teaspoons (10 ml) of nut butter or eat some raw vegetables with hummus. If feelings of hunger are triggered by emotions, explore ways you could respond differently to emotional challenges. For example, if sadness triggers the urge to eat, talk to someone or write in your journal. If stress triggers your hunger, go for a long walk, take a yoga class, or have a bubble bath. If anger triggers your hunger, write a letter to the editor, take it out on a punching bag, or a stomp around the block. If your hunger is linked to environmental stimulants, such as the doughnuts a coworker brought to the office, do what you can to transform your environment. Challenge your colleagues to bring in nutritious snacks and lead the charge by sharing healthy treats, such as kale chips or fresh fruit.

Nutritional Analyses: The nutrient values provided for the recipes in this book are estimates only, calculated from the individual ingredients used in each recipe based on the nutrition data found for those ingredients. Analyses do not include optional ingredients, garnishes, fat used to oil pans, or suggested accompaniments unless specific amounts are given.

Get Cooking with Whole Plant Foods

3

If you're not used to cooking beans, grains, and vegetables—or doing any cooking from scratch—this chapter will help you get started on your new adventure. Even if you've loved to cook for years, you might be unfamiliar with how to prepare beans and intact whole grains. If that's the case, be sure to check out the special sections on cooking beans (page 53) and cooking grains (page 54). These handy guides will be your go-to references throughout your plant-based cooking experience. If you keep cooked beans, cooked grains, and dark leafy greens in your fridge, you'll have the makings for an instant, healthy meal.

Most of the recipes in this book can be doubled, which makes it easy to prepare extras that can be used for another meal. Store leftovers in bulk or in individual portions. Legume-based soups and entrees freeze particularly well. Glass containers with lids are perfect for storing foods in the fridge or freezer.

Being organized will help you avoid having to switch pots and pans as you make a recipe or prevent you from being halfway into recipe prep before you realize you're missing a key ingredient. Our advice is to follow these steps to ensure success:

1. Read the recipe completely before starting.

2. Gather all the equipment and ingredients you'll need.

3. Set up the counter space. Arrange and organize the ingredients and equipment according to which items you'll use first. If you're short on counter space, bringing in a small portable table or island on wheels can instantly expand your work surface.

Equipment to Support Your Success

Consider kitchen equipment an investment in your health. Working with high-quality equipment will boost your confidence and capability and increase your motivation to perform the tasks at hand.

For starters, learn how to wield a chef's knife with ease. Sometimes people balk at eating fresh vegetables and fruits because of the preparation involved, such as having to peel, slice, dice, or chop. Inexpensive manual and electric food processors can take over some of this work, but often they don't give you much control over the size and thickness of the cuts—and you'll have to disassemble and wash an extra piece of equipment.

The most versatile way to prepare produce is by hand with an eight- or ten-inch chef's knife. You'll want one that feels balanced when you hold it by the handle and isn't so heavy that it's tiresome to use. If you have the time and resources to attend a local cooking class, you'll pick up great tips on how to prepare various vegetables. If classes aren't available locally, a quick search online will direct you to numerous videos on how to select a good knife, keep it sharpened (for your safety as well as for efficient use), and prepare different fruits and vegetables.

It's well worth the investment of a little time to improve your knife skills. The more you practice this skill, the better you'll get at it. You'll save money buying produce that's fresh and whole instead of packaged and prepared, and you'll be inclined to include a wider variety of produce in your diet if you can prepare it efficiently.

Following is a basic inventory of the tools you'll need to prepare all the recipes in this book, although you may want to begin with just a few of these items and add more to your collection once you gain experience.

COOKING UTENSILS

- Baking dishes, 13 x 9-inch (33 x 23 cm) and 8-inch (20-cm) square
- Baking sheets, 2
- Loaf pans, medium (6-cup/1.5 L capacity)
- Muffin pan, standard 12-cup (metal or silicone)
- Nonstick saucepan, medium
- Nonstick skillets, small and medium
- Saucepans with lids, 1–1½ quart (1–1.5 L), 2–3 quart (2–3 L), 4 quart (4 L)
- Soup pot with lid, 12 quart (36 L)
- Steamer basket

ELECTRIC APPLIANCES

- Blender
- Food processor
- Slow cooker or multipurpose pressure cooker and slow cooker (such as an Instant Pot)

HANDHELD TOOLS

- Can opener
- Garlic press
- Pancake turner (metal spatula)
- Rubber or silicone spatulas, small, medium, and large
- Slotted spoon
- Soup ladle
- Spring-loaded tongs
- Vegetable peeler
- Vegetable scrub brush
- Whisks, small and medium
- Wooden spoons, 2

KNIVES

- Chef's knife, 8 or 10 inch (20 or 25 cm)
- Paring knife

MISCELLANEOUS

- Colander
- Cutting boards, large and small
- Food grater
- Funnels, small and medium
- Measuring-cup set
- Measuring-spoon set
- Mixing bowls, 2 quart (2 L), 3 quart (3 L), 4 quart (4 L)
- Parchment paper or silicone baking mat

STORAGE ITEMS

- Canisters and jars for storing grains, dried legumes, and other dry goods
- Glass freezer containers
- Storage containers in a variety of sizes, with lids

Shopping List

The following shopping list is a convenient resource that itemizes both the staples used in the recipes in this book and the ingredients that may be used only occasionally or for recipe variations. **The ingredients shown in bold are used frequently throughout the recipes in chapter 4.** Start by purchasing these, and then buy other ingredients that are specific to the recipes you'd like to try.

You might want to photocopy this list so you can take it to the store with you when you go shopping. Feel free to customize it and include additional items of your own. Buy fresh produce in season as needed. Dry ingredients can be purchased in the appropriate amounts and stored indefinitely in sealed containers in a cool, dry place. For the best prices, look for sources that offer grains and legumes in bulk. Specialty stores that feature international foods and the international sections of supermarkets and natural food stores are often good places to find unfamiliar ingredients. See the recommendations on page 14 for purchasing organic produce.

VEGETABLES (FRESH)

Arugula

Asparagus

Avocados

Beans (green, yellow)

Beets (purple, yellow)

Bell peppers (green, orange, red, yellow)

Broccoli

Broccolini

Brussels sprouts

Cabbage (Chinese, green, napa, red/purple)

Carrots (orange, purple, yellow)

Cauliflower

Celery

Chives

Corn (fresh, frozen)

Cucumbers

Garlic

Ginger

Greens (beet, bok choy, collard, kale, mustard, spinach, turnip)

Kohlrabi

Jalapeño chile

Jicama

Lettuce (dark green, red)

Mushrooms

Onions (green, red, white, yellow)

Parsley

Parsnips

Peas (green, snow, sugar snap)

Potatoes

Pumpkins

Radicchio

Radishes (red, watermelon)

Rutabagas

Sprouts (alfalfa, broccoli, lentil, mung, pea, sunflower)

Sweet potatoes

Tomatoes (cherry, salad)

Turnips (young)

Watercress

Winter squash

Yams

Zucchini

(Commonly used items are in bold.)

FRUITS (FRESH, FROZEN, OR CANNED)

Apples

Applesauce (unsweetened)

Apricots

Bananas

Blackberries

Blueberries

Cherries

Cranberries

Grapefruits

Grapes

Lemons

Limes

Mangoes

Nectarines

Oranges

Papayas

Peaches

Pears, fresh and canned (unsweetened)

Pineapples

Plums

Pomegranates

Raspberries

Strawberries

FRUITS (DRIED, UNSWEETENED)

Apricots

Cherries

Coconut (unsweetened shredded dried)

Currants

Dates

Mangoes

Peaches

Pears

Prunes

Raisins (dark, golden)

GRAINS AND GRAIN PRODUCTS

Barley, whole grain (hulled, pot, Scotch)

Buckwheat groats

Cornmeal, whole grain (coarsely ground)

Kamut berries

Oat groats

Oats, rolled (old-fashioned)

Oats, steel cut

Quinoa

Rice (black, brown, brown basmati, red)

Spelt berries

Wild rice

LEGUMES (DRIED OR CANNED)

Adzuki beans

Black beans

Black-eyed peas

Cannellini beans

Chickpeas

Great Northern beans

Kidney beans (red, white)

Lentils (green, red, small brown or black)

Lima beans

Mung beans

Navy beans

Pink beans

Pinto beans

Red beans

Split peas (green, yellow)

White beans

NONDAIRY ALTERNATIVES

Nondairy milk, fortified and unsweetened (almond, cashew, hemp, rice, soy)

Nondairy yogurt, unsweetened

(Commonly used items are in bold.)

NUTS, SEEDS, BUTTERS

Almond butter

Almonds

Brazil nuts

Cashews

Chia seeds

Flaxseeds (whole or ground)

Hazelnuts

Hemp seeds

Macadamia nuts

Peanut butter

Pecans

Pumpkin seeds

Sesame seeds

Sunflower seeds

Tahini

Walnuts

HERBS AND SPICES

Allspice (ground)

Basil (dried, fresh)

Bay leaves

Cardamom (ground)

Cayenne

Celery seeds

Chili powder

Cilantro (fresh)

Cinnamon (ground, Ceylon)

Cloves (ground, whole)

Cumin (ground)

Dill (dried, fresh)

Garlic powder

Ginger (ground)

Marjoram (dried, fresh)

Mint (dried, fresh)

Mustard, dry

Nutmeg (grated or ground)

Onion powder

Oregano

Paprika (smoked, sweet)

Parsley (dried, fresh)

Pepper, black (ground)

Poultry seasoning

Pumpkin pie spice

Red pepper flakes (crushed)

Rosemary (dried, fresh)

Salt

Savory (dried, fresh)

Tarragon (dried, fresh)

Thyme (dried)

Turmeric (ground)

MISCELLANEOUS ITEMS

Arrowroot starch

Baking powder

Baking soda

Bragg Liquid Aminos

Cocoa or cacao powder (unsweetened)

Cornstarch

Curry paste (Patak's mild)

Horseradish (prepared)

Miso (dark, light)

Mustard (Dijon, spicy brown, or stone-ground)

Nori sheets

Nutritional yeast flakes

Olives (black)

Red peppers (roasted)

Stevia

Tamari (reduced sodium)

Tempeh

Tofu (medium, firm, extra-firm)

Tomato paste

Tomatoes, canned (crushed, diced)

Tomatoes, sun-dried

Vanilla extract

Vegetable broth (cubes, liquid, powder)

Vinegar (balsamic, cider)

(Commonly used items are in bold.)

Cooking Legumes

I t's both practical and economical to cook legumes in quantity so you'll have different types on hand whenever you want them. Freeze individual or meal-sized portions of cooked legumes in labeled ziplock bags or glass jars for as long as six months.

One option is to invest in a slow cooker, pressure cooker, or multi-use programmable pressure cooker and follow the instructions that accompany it for cooking legumes. If you prefer to cook beans on the stove top, the following are our recommendations:

1. Spread the dried legumes on a tray so you can easily see any small rocks, twigs, or other debris that might have come through the mechanical cleaning process. Rinse the legumes well to remove any dirt and put them in a large saucepan or soup pot.

2. Soaking legumes before cooking is essential for increasing digestibility. Lentils and split peas are the exceptions; they may be cooked without presoaking. However, if you have difficulty digesting them, you may notice an improvement if you soak those smaller legumes before cooking.

3. Add enough water to cover the dried legumes by at least one inch (3 cm), then cover the saucepan with a lid and soak the legumes for six to eight hours. Be sure to drain off the soaking water before cooking the legumes; in doing so, you'll discard some of the substances that contribute to flatulence and indigestibility. If you want to speed up the presoaking process, cover the legumes with fresh water, bring to a boil, and boil for one minute. Remove from the heat, cover, and let rest for at least one hour. Then discard the soaking water and proceed with cooking.

4. To cook, put unsoaked lentils and split peas or drained and rinsed larger legumes in a large saucepan with a tight-fitting lid. Add the amount of water indicated in table 7 (page 54), bring to a boil, then decrease the heat and simmer for the time indicated. During cooking, skim off any foam that rises to the top, as dissolved substances in the foam can also cause flatulence. The beans are done when you can soften them on the roof of your mouth with your tongue. At this stage, they're the most digestible.

TABLE 7 Cooking legumes

DRIED LEGUMES (1 CUP/250 ML)	PRESOAK	COOKING WATER	COOKING TIMES for lentils, split peas, and soaked beans*	APPROXIMATE YIELD
Adzuki beans, black beans, black-eyed peas, cannellini beans	Yes	4 cups (1 L)	45–60 minutes	2½ cups (625 ml)
Great Northern beans, kidney beans, lima beans, navy beans, pink beans, pinto beans, red beans (small)	Yes	3 cups (750 ml)	1½–2 hours	2–2½ cups (500–625 ml)
Chickpeas	Yes	4 cups (1 L)	2–3 hours	2½ cups (625 ml)
Lentils (brown, gray, green)	No	3 cups (750 ml)	45 minutes	2¼ cups (550 ml)
Lentils, split (red)	No	3 cups (750 ml)	15–20 minutes	2¼ cups (550 ml)
Peas, split (green, yellow)	No	3 cups (750 ml)	30–45 minutes	2¼ cups (550 ml)

*Beans that are large or old or have been stored for long periods of time will take longer to cook.

By adding simple seasonings, such as garlic and onion (fresh or dried), during cooking, the beans will be quite flavorful when they're done. They can be served as is, without any additional preparation, on top of grains, starchy vegetables, or salads. Add acidic ingredients (such as vinegar, chopped tomatoes, or tomato juice) near the end of the cooking time, when the beans are just tender. If these ingredients are added sooner, they can make the beans tough and slow the cooking process.

Cooking Grains

It will be easier to add small amounts of whole grains to soups, salads, and meals if you cook large quantities of them at a time. You can store individual or meal-sized portions of cooked grains in the freezer in labeled ziplock bags or glass jars; they will keep for six months.

Cook whole grains in a heavy saucepan with a tight-fitting lid to retain moisture. Bring the amount of water recommended in table 8 (page 56) to a boil over medium-high heat. Add the grain, stir, and return to a boil. Decrease the heat to low, cover, and cook for the recommended time. Many

SODIUM SMARTS

The menus and recipes in this book have been designed to provide a total of less than 1,500 mg of sodium per day. This is a suitable level of intake for people with diabetes, heart disease, or high blood pressure.

To further reduce the sodium content of recipes:

- Omit added salt or reduce the amount and add it near the end of cooking.
- When there are a number of salty seasoning options (such as Bragg Liquid Aminos, miso, salt, soy sauce, or tamari), choose the one with the lowest amount of sodium, reduce amount used (for example, cut the amount in half), or omit this ingredient altogether. Some of these salty seasonings offer lower-sodium versions. For example, reduced-sodium tamari has about 25 percent less sodium than regular tamari. Cutting the amount of regular tamari in half would result in a greater sodium reduction than using reduced-sodium tamari.
- Check labels on jarred and canned foods. Choose salt-free or low-sodium products.
- Use salt-free or low-sodium vegetable broth or replace the broth with water.

To boost flavor without adding sodium:

- Increase the amounts of herbs and seasonings.
- Add a squeeze of lemon or lime juice to the finished dish.

whole grains will fluff up if you remove the saucepan from the heat after the grain is cooked and let it rest covered for a few minutes. This will also help the individual grains separate and not stick together as much when leftovers are stored.

If the cooked grain has stuck to the bottom of the saucepan, remove the pan from the heat, add a very small amount of water or other liquid, cover the pan, and let the grain sit for a few minutes. It will loosen, making it easier to serve the grain and clean the saucepan.

TABLE 8 Cooking grains

GRAIN, UNCOOKED (1 CUP/250 ML)	COOKING WATER	COOKING TIME	APPROXIMATE YIELD
Barley, hulled (whole grain, pot, or Scotch)	3½ cups (875 ml)	1 hour	3½ cups (875 ml)
Buckwheat groats	2 cups (500 ml)	20 minutes	3 cups (750 ml)
Kamut berries	3 cups (750 ml)	70–80 minutes (60 minutes if soaked in advance for 8–10 hours)	3 cups (750 ml)
Oats, steel cut	4 cups (1 L)	20 minutes	4 cups (1 L)
Quinoa (any color)	2 cups (500 ml)	15 minutes (let stand covered for 5 minutes after cooking)	3 cups (750 ml)
Rice, brown (brown basmati, long grain, short grain)*	5 cups (1,250 ml)	40–50 minutes, then drain	3½ cups (875 ml)
Spelt berries or oat groats	3 cups (750 ml)	45–60 minutes	2½ cups (625 ml)
Wild rice	3 cups (750 ml)	40–45 minutes (let stand covered for 10 minutes after cooking)	3½–4 cups (875 ml–1 L)

*Although rice is commonly cooked using 2 cups (500 ml) water per 1 cup (250 ml) rice, this method helps to reduce arsenic content by about 50 percent. Soaking the rice for 8–12 hours and draining prior to cooking cuts cooking time in half and reduces arsenic by about 80 percent.

A NOTE ABOUT SWEETENERS

Dates are used as the primary sweetener in most of the recipes in this book. In contrast to added sugars, which have a lot of calories but no fiber and very few nutrients, dates are loaded with fiber and are a rich source of magnesium, potassium, and B vitamins, especially vitamin B_6. They also have a relatively low glycemic index, ranging from 44 to 54.

The most common dates sold in North America are deglet noor (small, dry, firm dates) and medjool (large, moist, sweet dates). There are well over one hundred varieties of dates, and they are all suitable for these recipes. If the dates you have are hard and dry, they can be softened by steaming them or soaking them in boiling water for a few minutes, then draining. Steaming is preferable because nutrients and flavor will be lost in the soaking water. To preserve their freshness, freeze dates when you purchase them in volume and refrigerate only what you will use within a month or two.

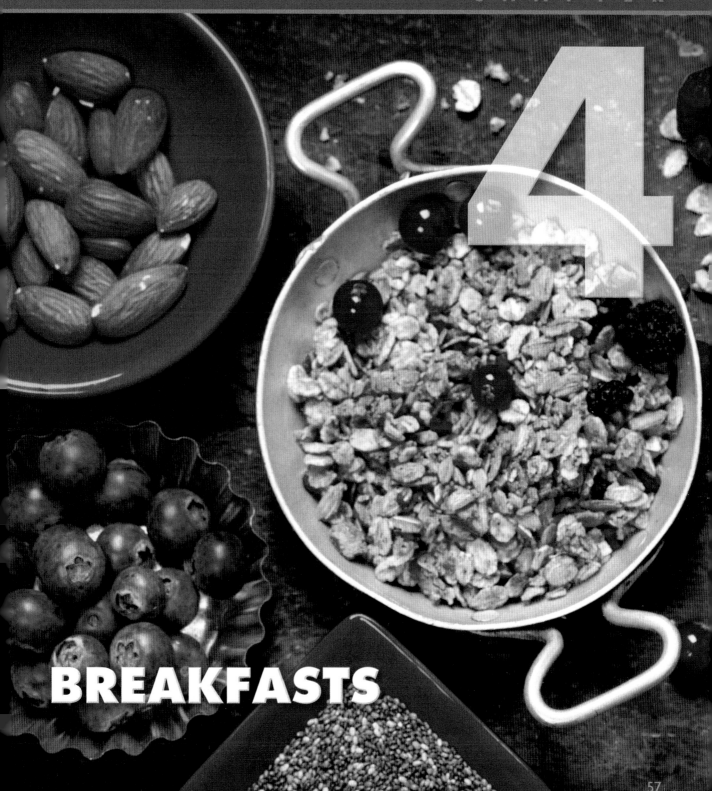

4

BREAKFASTS

Simple Morning Muesli

MAKES 2 CUPS
(500 ML),
2 SERVINGS

This nourishing breakfast can be prepared the night before and provides an excellent balance of protein, fat, and carbohydrate. Soaking enhances the digestibility of the grains and increases mineral absorption. One cup (250 ml) provides 12 grams of protein and 8 grams of fiber.

Store nuts and seeds in the freezer to preserve their freshness. For convenience, mix your favorite nut-and-seed combination in a single jar.

¾ cup (185 ml) old-fashioned rolled oats or other rolled grains

2 tablespoons (30 ml) raisins or other dried fruit

2 tablespoons (30 ml) chopped walnuts, almonds, or other nuts

¼ teaspoon (1 ml) ground cinnamon

1 cup (250 ml) fortified unsweetened soy milk or other nondairy milk

1 cup (250 ml) fresh fruit (such as blueberries or chopped apple, mango, or peach)

1 tablespoon (15 ml) ground flaxseeds or chia seeds

Put the oats, raisins, walnuts, cinnamon, milk, and fresh fruit in a medium glass or ceramic bowl and stir to combine. Refrigerate for 8–10 hours. Alternatively, stir in the fresh fruit just before serving to preserve its color and nutrition. Top with the flaxseeds just before serving.

VARIATION: Replace some of the soy milk with nondairy yogurt.

Per serving:
(1 cup/250 ml):
calories: 312
protein: 10 g
fat: 11 g
carbohydrate: 47 g
dietary fiber: 8 g
calcium: 229 mg
sodium: 51 mg

Note: Analysis done with blueberries.

MAKING PLANT MILKS MORE NUTRITIOUS

Always choose fortified (enriched) unsweetened nondairy milks. Among nondairy beverages, soy milk is significantly higher in protein. To boost the protein, vitamins, and minerals of 1 quart (1 L) of any nondairy beverage, blend 2 cups (500 ml) of the milk with ⅓–½ cup (85–125 ml) of hemp seeds until very smooth. If you use a high-speed blender, this will take one to two minutes. Pour the blended milk back into the container and shake well. Store in the refrigerator.

Sweet Breakfast Bowl

Brimming with nutrients, antioxidants, and fiber, this breakfast will keep you satisfied all morning long. Once the ingredients have been gathered, it comes together in a flash. Begin with cooked whole grain, then add your favorite toppings. For a takeout breakfast, layer the ingredients in a mason jar. Below are suggestions to get you started. Use as much or as little of a component as you like, depending on how hungry you are.

Whole Grains (½–1 cup/125–250 ml)

- Cooked hulled or pot barley, Kamut berries, oat groats, steel-cut oats, or spelt berries

Fruit. *Fresh or thawed frozen fruit, stewed fruit, or both*

- Fresh berries; chopped apples, apricots, nectarines, peaches, or other fresh or thawed frozen fruit (1 cup/250 ml)
- Stewed fruit, without added sugar, such as applesauce, berries, prunes, or plums (¼–½ cup/60–125 ml)

Nuts/Seeds (1 tablespoon/15 ml). *Choose 1 omega-3-rich seed and one other*

- Omega-3-rich seeds (chia, flax, hemp)
- Other seeds (pumpkin, sunflower)
- Nuts (chopped almonds, Brazil nuts, hazelnuts, pecans, or walnuts)

Optional Creamy Additions (2–4 tablespoons/30–60 ml)

- Cashew-Pear Cream (page 171)
- Unsweetened nondairy yogurt
- Vanilla Chia Pudding (page 162)

Fortified Unsweetened Soy Milk or Other Nondairy Milk (½–1 cup/ 125–250 ml)

Optional Spices (¼–½ teaspoon/1–2 ml)

- Ground allspice, cardamom, cinnamon, cloves, nutmeg, or pumpkin pie spice

Put all the ingredients in a bowl and stir until well combined.

Store nuts and seeds in the freezer to preserve their freshness. For convenience, mix your favorite nut-and-seed combination in a single jar.

Wholly Granola

MAKES 7 CUPS
(1.75 L),
14 SERVINGS

Granolas are notoriously high in oil and sugar, but this one is oil- and sugar-free! It gets its sweetness from fruit and its fat from nuts and seeds. Serve it with unsweetened nondairy milk or yogurt or Vanilla Chia Pudding (page 162) and fresh fruit.

2 tablespoons (30 ml) **water**

¼ cup (60 ml) **pitted soft dates** (about 8 dates)

¼ cup (60 ml) **nut or seed butter**

½ **banana**

½ **orange, peeled and seeded; or ½ apple, cored; or 3 tablespoons** (45 ml) **water**

1½ teaspoons (7 ml) **ground cinnamon**

1 teaspoon (5 ml) **vanilla extract**

3 cups (750 ml) **old-fashioned rolled oats**

1 cup (250 ml) **sunflower, pumpkin, or chia seeds, or a combination**

½ cup (125 ml) **coarsely chopped almonds or other nuts**

¼ cup (60 ml) **unsweetened shredded dried coconut** (optional)

⅓ cup (85 ml) **dried currants or raisins** (optional)

This granola also makes an excellent dessert served with fresh fruit and Cashew-Pear Cream (page 171). Double the recipe to cut time in the kitchen. Storing it in the freezer will help keep it crisp and fresh.

Preheat the oven to 250 degrees F (120 degrees C). Line two baking sheets with parchment paper or silicone baking mats.

Put the water, dates, nut butter, banana, orange, cinnamon, and vanilla extract in a blender or food processor and process into a smooth paste.

Put the oats, sunflower seeds, almonds, and optional coconut in a large bowl and stir to combine. Add the paste and stir until well combined. Spread equally on the lined baking sheets. Bake for 1 hour, stirring halfway through the baking time. If the granola isn't quite dry after an hour, turn off the oven and let it rest in the oven for an additional hour until dry.

Transfer to a large bowl and stir in the optional currants. Stored in sealed containers or ziplock freezer bags in the freezer, the granola will keep for 3 months.

Per serving
(½ cup/125 ml):
calories: 222
protein: 7 g
fat: 12 g
carbohydrate: 24 g
dietary fiber: 5 g
calcium: 46 mg
sodium: 7 mg

Savory Steel-Cut Oats

MAKES 5 CUPS
(1.25 L),
4 SERVINGS

Here's a tasty twist on standard steel-cut oats. It makes an enticing breakfast for people who prefer savory over sweet. If you have a slow cooker, this recipe can cook overnight while you sleep and will be hot and ready when you wake up. Simply omit the greens and add them in the morning.

3 cups (750 ml) water or vegetable broth

1 cup (250 ml) diced onion

1 cup (250 ml) chopped mushrooms

1 cup (250 ml) steel-cut oats

1 small red bell pepper, chopped

2 tablespoons (30 ml) reduced-sodium tamari (optional)

1 clove garlic, crushed (optional)

1 teaspoon (5 ml) dried herbs (such as basil, oregano, thyme, savory, tarragon, or turmeric; optional)

2 cups (500 ml) stemmed and chopped dark leafy greens (such as collard greens or kale), **packed**

1 cup (250 ml) cooked or canned beans (any kind), **drained and rinsed**

Freshly ground black pepper (optional)

Store leftovers in the refrigerator and heat up just the amount you need.

Put the water, onion, mushrooms, oats, bell pepper, optional tamari, optional garlic, and optional herbs in a large saucepan and stir to combine. Bring to a boil over medium-high heat, decrease the heat to low, cover, and cook for 25 minutes. Stir in the greens and beans and cook, stirring frequently, until heated through and the greens have softened, 2–3 minutes. Season with pepper to taste if desired. Serve hot.

VARIATIONS: For added protein and crunch, sprinkle the cooked oats with chopped nuts or hemp, pumpkin, sesame, or sunflower seeds just before serving. For added flavor and texture, top with chopped fresh herbs (such as cilantro or parsley), chopped green onions, nutritional yeast, or sprouts.

Per serving
(1¼ cups/310 ml):
calories: 249
protein: 12 g
fat: 3 g
carbohydrate: 48 g
dietary fiber: 6 g
calcium: 178 mg
sodium: 19 mg

Note: Analysis done with basil, collard greens, and black beans.

Barley and Oat Groat Porridge

MAKES 4 CUPS
(1 L), 3 SERVINGS

This makes a substantial morning meal with a pleasant variety of textures and flavors. Of all the whole grains, barley has the lowest glycemic index and is brimming with soluble fiber, so it's especially helpful for people with diabetes.

If you enjoy having handy leftovers, make a double batch, store the extras in the fridge, and serve hot or cold for breakfast throughout the week.

4 cups (1 L) water

½ cup (125 ml) hulled or pot barley

½ cup (125 ml) oat groats, Kamut berries, or spelt berries

¼ teaspoon (1 ml) salt (optional)

¾ cup (185 ml) fortified unsweetened soy milk or other nondairy milk, plus more as needed

¼ cup (60 ml) raisins, dried currants, or other chopped dried fruit (such as apricots, peaches, pears, or prunes)

Put the water, barley, oat groats, and optional salt in a large saucepan. Bring to a simmer over medium-high heat. Decrease the heat to medium-low and cook, stirring occasionally, until the water is absorbed and the oats are tender, 1–1½ hours. Stir in the milk and raisins and cook for 15 minutes longer. If the porridge is too thick, add more milk or water as desired.

PRESSURE-COOKER PORRIDGE: Put the barley, oat groats, and salt in a pressure cooker. Add the recommended amount of water for grains for your particular cooker and proceed according to the manufacturer's directions. Add milk and raisins when serving.

SLOW-COOKER PORRIDGE: Put the barley, oat groats, water, and salt in a slow cooker and cook for 8–10 hours on the lowest setting. Stir in the milk and raisins shortly before serving.

Per serving
(1⅓ cups/325 ml):
calories: 307
protein: 11 g
fat: 4 g
carbohydrate: 59 g
dietary fiber: 9 g
calcium: 84 mg
sodium: 34 mg

Baked Apple-Spice Oatmeal

MAKES 4½ CUPS
(1.125 L),
4 SERVINGS

Baked oatmeal is a welcome comfort food, plus it's rich in soluble fiber, vitamins, minerals, antioxidants, and phytochemicals. Although intact whole grains are generally best, this is a lovely dish to add variety to your repertoire or to serve to company. It also freezes beautifully.

1¼ cups (310 ml) **old-fashioned rolled oats or steel-cut oats**

2 apples, diced

¼ cup (60 ml) **walnuts, chopped**

¼ cup (60 ml) **raisins, currants, or chopped prunes or other dried fruit**

2 tablespoons (30 ml) **raw sunflower seeds**

2 tablespoons (30 ml) **unsweetened shredded dried coconut**

1½ teaspoons (7 ml) **ground cinnamon, plus more for sprinkling**

¼ teaspoon (1 ml) **ground cloves**

2 cups (500 ml) **fortified unsweetened soy milk or other nondairy milk,**
    plus more for serving

1 teaspoon (5 ml) **vanilla extract**

¼ teaspoon (1 ml) **salt** (optional)

Ground flaxseeds or chia seeds (optional)

Preheat the oven to 375 degrees F (190 degrees C).

Put the oats, apples, walnuts, raisins, sunflower seeds, coconut, cinnamon, and cloves in a deep 7-inch (18-cm) or 8-inch (20-cm) square baking dish. Put the milk, vanilla extract, and optional salt in a small bowl and whisk to combine. Pour over the oat mixture and stir to combine. Sprinkle with additional cinnamon. Bake for 45 minutes, or until the top is lightly browned. Serve with additional milk and a sprinkling of flaxseeds if desired.

VARIATIONS: Add ground allspice, cardamom, or nutmeg to taste. Replace the apples with 2 pears or bananas or 1½ cups (375 ml) blueberries. Double the recipe for a crowd (or if you want leftovers) and use a 13 x 9-inch (33 x 23-cm) baking pan.

Per serving:
calories: 302
protein: 9 g
fat: 12 g
carbohydrate: 43 g
dietary fiber: 7 g
calcium: 226 mg
sodium: 53 mg

Beans, Greens, and Sweet Potato with Tahini-Lime Sauce

MAKES 3 CUPS
(750 ML),
2 SERVINGS

Simple and satisfying, this dish is an appetizing way to start the day. For even more antioxidant power and savory flavor, add minced garlic, diced red onion, grated ginger, or ground turmeric to the sauce.

TAHINI-LIME SAUCE

¼ **cup (60 ml) tahini**

1 **tablespoon (15 ml) lime juice, plus more as needed**

2 **teaspoons (10 ml) tamari**

¼ **cup (60 ml) water, plus more as needed**

BEANS, GREENS, AND SWEET POTATO

1 **orange sweet potato, peeled and cubed**

3 **cups (750 ml) chopped dark leafy greens** (see Tip), **packed**

1 **cup (250 ml) cooked or canned black beans, drained and rinsed**

Freshly ground black pepper

To make the sauce, put the tahini in a small bowl. Add the lime juice and tamari and stir with a fork to combine. Add the water and additional lime juice to achieve the desired tartness and consistency.

To prepare the beans, greens, and sweet potato, steam the sweet potato for 10 minutes. Add the greens and steam until just wilted, about 3 minutes. Add the beans and steam until heated through, about 2 minutes. Transfer to a medium bowl and season with pepper to taste. Serve hot with the sauce on the side.

Per serving
(1½ cups/375 ml):
calories: 382
protein: 16 g
fat: 17 g
carbohydrate: 47 g
dietary fiber: 13 g
calcium: 156 mg
sodium: 379 mg

Note: Analysis done with kale.

For the greens, use bok choy or stemmed kale, collard greens, or spinach. Alternatively, use Brussels sprouts and add them with the sweet potato since they'll take longer to cook. If you double the recipe, increase the water or broth for the beans, greens, and sweet potatoes by only ¼ cup (60 ml) to keep the mixture from becoming too watery.

Golden Scrambled Tofu and Veggies

njoy this protein-rich dish for breakfast, lunch, or dinner. If you like, serve it with salsa, diced avocado, cooked sweet potatoes, or leftover vegetables mixed in or spooned on top. Alternatively, serve a slice of dense pumpernickel bread on the side.

MAKES 2½–3 CUPS
(625–750 ML),
2 SERVINGS

1 package (12–16 ounces/350–450 g) **firm or medium-firm tofu, drained**

1 teaspoon (5 ml) **tamari**

½ teaspoon (2 ml) **ground turmeric**

¼ cup (60 ml) **sliced green onion, or 1 teaspoon** (5 ml) **onion powder**

2 cloves **garlic, crushed, or 1 teaspoon** (5 ml) **garlic powder**

2 tablespoons (30 ml) **water or vegetable broth, plus more as needed**

2 cups (500 ml) **finely chopped dark leafy greens** (see Tip), **packed**

1 cup (250 ml) **chopped mushrooms**

½ cup (125 ml) **diced red bell pepper**

2 tablespoons (30 ml) **nutritional yeast flakes**

For the greens, select from bok choy or stemmed kale, collard greens, spinach, or parsley. If you use tender greens, such as spinach or parsley, add them during the last 5 minutes of cooking.

Crumble the tofu into a medium bowl. For a finer texture, mash it with a fork. Add the tamari and turmeric and stir until evenly distributed. Add the onion powder and garlic powder, if using, and stir to combine.

Put the water in a large nonstick skillet. If you don't have a nonstick skillet, mist a regular skillet with cooking spray. Add the green onion and garlic, if using, and the greens, mushrooms, and bell pepper. Cook over medium heat, stirring occasionally, until the vegetables are soft, about 5 minutes. Add a little more water if the vegetables start to stick. Add the tofu and cook, stirring frequently, until the water has evaporated and the tofu is hot. The consistency should resemble scrambled eggs. If the tofu sticks or gets dried out, add a little more water as needed. Remove from the heat and stir in the nutritional yeast (if added earlier, it will stick to the pan). Serve hot.

Per serving:
calories: 214
protein: 23 g
fat: 10 g
carbohydrate: 13 g
dietary fiber: 5 g
calcium: 514 mg
sodium: 229 mg

Note: Analysis done with calcium-set tofu and kale.

Banana-Walnut Pancakes

MAKES 10 SMALL
PANCAKES,
5 SERVINGS

These dense, hearty pancakes have a fabulous flavor. They rise best when the batter is spread thin. Top them with fruit, nut butter, or Very Berry Sauce (page 170), or try a combination of all three.

1½ cups (375 ml) **old-fashioned rolled oats**

3 tablespoons (45 ml) **ground flaxseeds**

1½ teaspoons (7 ml) **baking powder**

1 teaspoon (5 ml) **ground cinnamon**

¼ teaspoon (1 ml) **salt** (optional)

⅛ teaspoon (0.5 ml) **ground cloves or nutmeg** (optional)

2 ripe bananas, **broken into pieces**

1 cup (250 ml) **fortified unsweetened soy milk or other nondairy milk**

⅓ cup (85 ml) **coarsely chopped walnuts**

Put the oats, flaxseeds, baking powder, cinnamon, optional salt, and optional cloves in a food processor and process until the consistency of flour. Add the bananas and milk and process until smooth. Add the walnuts and pulse just until evenly incorporated.

Heat a large nonstick skillet over medium heat until hot enough that drops of water dance across it. If you don't have a nonstick skillet, mist a regular skillet with cooking spray. Use about ¼ cup (60 ml) of batter per pancake. Cook the pancakes in small batches; don't crowd them in the skillet. About three pancakes will fit in one large skillet. Spread the batter with a silicone spatula so the pancakes aren't too thick. Cook until the pancakes are lightly browned on the bottom, 2–3 minutes. Flip the pancakes over and cook the other side until lightly browned, about 2 minutes.

Per 2 pancakes:
calories: 238
protein: 8 g
fat: 9 g
carbohydrate: 33 g
dietary fiber: 7 g
calcium: 213 mg
sodium: 132 mg

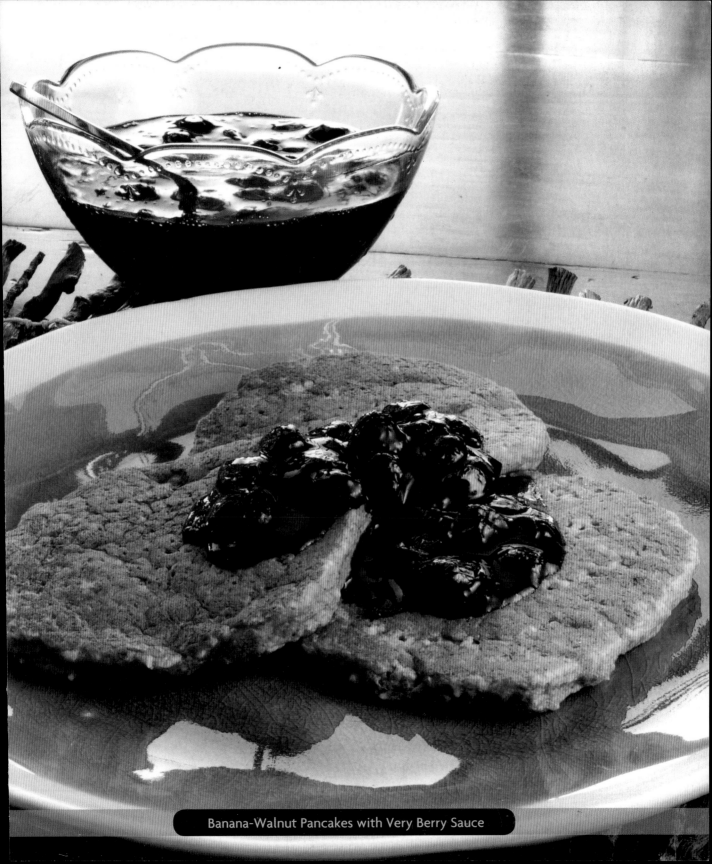

Banana-Walnut Pancakes with Very Berry Sauce

Carrot Spice Muffins

MAKES 12 MUFFINS

These tender muffins are mildly sweet and packed with great nutrition. Because the batter is prepared in a blender, it's quick and easy to make. Serve the muffins fresh from the oven or at room temperature, plain or with a little nut or seed butter.

- 2 cups (500 ml) **old-fashioned rolled oats**
- ¼ cup (60 ml) **ground flaxseeds**
- 2 teaspoons (10 ml) **ground cinnamon**
- 1½ teaspoons (7 ml) **baking powder**
- ½ teaspoon (2 ml) **baking soda**
- ½ teaspoon (2 ml) **salt**
- ½ teaspoon (2 ml) **ground ginger**
- ¼ teaspoon (1 ml) **ground cloves**
- ¼ teaspoon (1 ml) **ground nutmeg**
- ¼ cup (60 ml) **hemp seeds**

- 1½ cups (375 ml) **fortified unsweetened soy milk or other non-dairy milk**
- 3 medium or 2 large **carrots, chopped**
- 1 **apple, diced**
- ½ cup (125 ml) **pitted soft dates**
- 1 tablespoon (15 ml) **apple cider vinegar**
- 1 teaspoon (5 ml) **vanilla extract**
- ½ cup (125 ml) **coarsely chopped walnuts**
- ⅓ cup (85 ml) **raisins**

Preheat the oven to 375 degrees F (190 degrees C). Oil a standard twelve-cup muffin pan or mist it with cooking spray. Alternatively, use a silicone muffin pan.

Put the oats, flaxseeds, cinnamon, baking powder, baking soda, salt, ginger, cloves, and nutmeg in a blender and process until the consistency of flour. Transfer to a large bowl.

Put the hemp seeds and milk in the blender and process until creamy. Add the carrots, apple, dates, vinegar, and vanilla extract. Pulse just until well combined but not smooth (there should be some texture). Pour into the oat mixture and stir just until combined. Fold in the walnuts and raisins.

Spoon the batter evenly into the prepared muffin pan. Bake for 20–25 minutes, until a toothpick inserted in the center of a muffin comes out clean. Let cool in the pan on a cooling rack, then remove from the muffin cups using a table knife.

Per muffin:
calories: 179
protein: 5 g
fat: 7 g
carbohydrate: 25 g
dietary fiber: 5 g
calcium: 122 mg
sodium: 219 mg

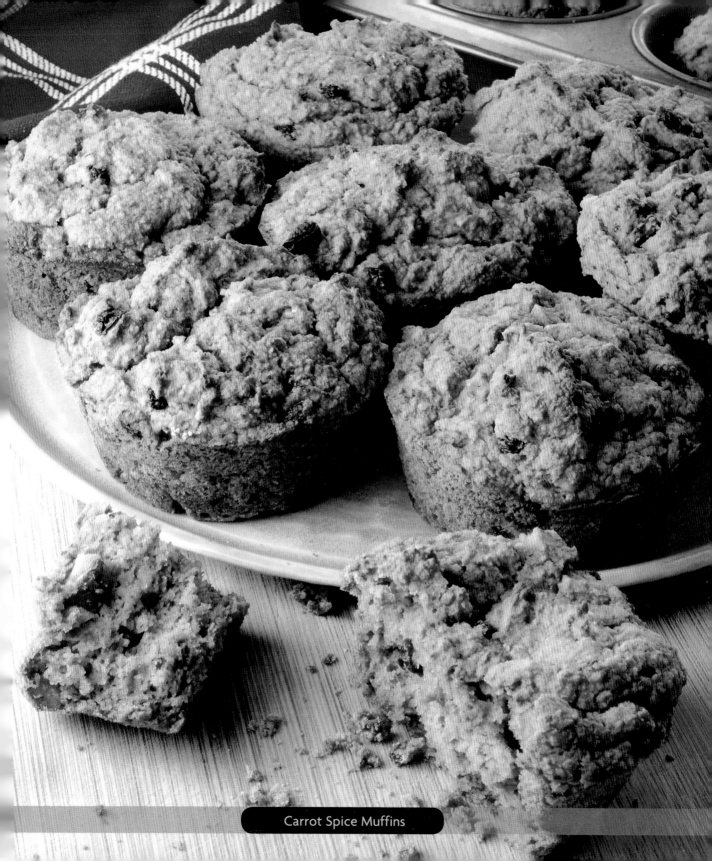

Carrot Spice Muffins

5

SOUPS

Better Broth Base

Most vegetable-broth powders and cubes are based on palm oil or other hard fats, sugar, salt, and flavorings. This tasty broth powder is based on B-vitamin-rich nutritional yeast and seasonings (salt can be reduced as desired for those who prefer a lower-sodium option). Keep a batch on hand to use in place of broth in soups and stews. Adjust the herbs and spices to suit your palate. If desired, reduce or omit the salt.

MAKES ABOUT 2 CUPS
(500 ML)

1 cup (250 ml) nutritional yeast flakes

½ cup (125 ml) dried onion flakes, or 3 tablespoons (45 ml) onion powder

2 tablespoons (30 ml) dried garlic flakes, or 1 tablespoon (15 ml) garlic powder

1 tablespoon (15 ml) salt

1 tablespoon (15 ml) dried oregano

1 tablespoon (15 ml) dried parsley flakes

1 teaspoon (5 ml) ground black pepper

1 teaspoon (5 ml) ground celery seeds

1 teaspoon (5 ml) paprika

1 teaspoon (5 ml) dried thyme

1 teaspoon (5 ml) ground turmeric

Put all the ingredients in a medium bowl and stir until well combined. Stored in an airtight container at room temperature, the broth base will keep for 3 months. To use, mix 1 tablespoon (15 ml) of broth base in 1 cup (250 ml) of boiling water.

Per 1 tablespoon (15 ml):
calories: 12
protein: 1 g
fat: 0 g
carbohydrate: 2 g
dietary fiber: 1 g
calcium: 8 mg
sodium: 237 mg

Green-Gold Cauliflower Soup

MAKES 7 CUPS
(1.75 L)

The combination of ingredients in this nutrient-packed soup creates a beautiful green-gold hue. Blended cashews make it rich and creamy, and nutritional yeast flakes contribute a boost of B-vitamins, including vitamin B_{12}.

4½ cups (1.125 L) **water**

1 onion, chopped

¼ cup (60 ml) **hulled or pot barley**

1 tablespoon (15 ml) **dried parsley flakes**

1¼ teaspoons (6 ml) **salt**

1 teaspoon (5 ml) **dried oregano**

1 teaspoon (5 ml) **whole celery seeds**

1 potato, peeled and diced

1 carrot, grated

1 stalk celery, finely chopped

2 cloves garlic, crushed

2 cups (500 ml) **small cauliflower florets**

1 cup (250 ml) **peas or small broccoli florets**

⅓ cup (85 ml) **raw cashews**

3 tablespoons (45 ml) **nutritional yeast flakes**

If you prefer a smooth soup, process it in batches in a blender. For a thinner soup, add additional water to achieve the desired consistency.

Put 4 cups (1 L) of the water and the onion, barley, parsley, salt, oregano, and celery seeds in a large soup pot and bring to a boil over medium-high heat. Decrease the heat to medium-low, cover, and simmer for 20 minutes. Add the potato, carrot, celery, and garlic. Cover and simmer until the vegetables are almost tender, 8–10 minutes. Add the cauliflower and peas, cover, and simmer until all the vegetables are tender, about 10 minutes.

Put the remaining ½ cup (125 ml) of water and the cashews in a blender and process until smooth. Add to the soup pot along with the nutritional yeast. Cook, stirring occasionally, until heated through.

Per 1 cup (250 ml):
calories: 122
protein: 5 g
fat: 3 g
carbohydrate: 20 g
dietary fiber: 5 g
calcium: 43 mg
sodium: 473 mg

Garden Blend Soup

MAKES 2½ CUPS
(625 ML)

Kale supplies more nutritional value per calorie than almost any other food. So keep the kale in this uncooked soup, but you can vary the other vegetables to suit your taste. Sunflower seeds are soaked prior to blending to increase the bioavailability of their minerals. In cooler months, use very hot water for a warm soup.

4 cups (1 L) stemmed and chopped kale, packed

½ orange, peeled, seeded, and coarsely chopped

½ apple, peeled if desired and chopped, or ½ small cucumber, peeled and chopped

¾ cup (185 ml) cold or hot water

¼ cup (60 ml) fresh herbs (such as basil, cilantro, dill, or parsley)**, packed**

1 tablespoon (15 ml) light miso

½ green onion, sliced (optional)

1½ teaspoons (7 ml) lemon juice

¼ red jalapeño chile with seeds, or pinch cayenne

½ clove garlic

¼ cup (60 ml) raw sunflower seeds, soaked for 1 hour, rinsed, and drained, or ½ avocado, coarsely chopped

¼ cup (60 ml) mung bean sprouts or pumpkin seeds, for garnish

Put the kale, orange, apple, water, herbs, miso, optional green onion, lemon juice, chile, and garlic in a blender and process until smooth. Add the sunflower seeds and process until smooth. Garnish with the sprouts. Serve immediately.

Per 1¼ cups (310 ml):
calories: 221
protein: 10 g
fat: 9 g
carbohydrate: 32 g
dietary fiber: 7 g
calcium: 237 mg
sodium: 431 mg

Note: Analysis done with basil and mung bean sprouts.

Kale and Avocado Soup

MAKES 4 CUPS
(1 L)

Two nutritional superstars are featured in this creamy blended soup—kale and avocado. Avocado is high in healthy fat and is a concentrated source of fiber and plant sterols. Part of the avocado is used as a garnish, but you can blend all of it if you prefer.

4 cups (1 L) **water or vegetable broth**

4 cups (1 L) **stemmed and chopped kale, packed**

1 small onion, chopped

1 stalk celery, chopped, or 1 cup (250 ml) **chopped zucchini**

3 cloves garlic, crushed

1 teaspoon (5 ml) **dried rosemary, crushed**

1 large avocado, cubed

2 tablespoons (30 ml) **lemon or lime juice**

½ teaspoon (2 ml) **salt (optional)**

Freshly ground black pepper

Put the water, kale, onion, celery, garlic, and rosemary in a medium saucepan and bring to a boil over medium-high heat. Cover, decrease the heat to medium, and cook, stirring occasionally, until the vegetables are tender, 20–25 minutes. Pour into a blender. Add half the avocado and all the lemon juice and process until smooth and creamy. Alternatively, use an immersion blender to process the soup directly in the saucepan. Add the optional salt and season with pepper to taste. If the soup is too thick, add more water to achieve the desired consistency. Garnish each serving with the remaining avocado. Serve immediately. Stored in a sealed container in the refrigerator, leftover soup will keep for 1 day.

Per 1 cup (250 ml):
calories: 129
protein: 4 g
fat: 8 g
carbohydrate: 15 g
dietary fiber: 5 g
calcium: 113 mg
sodium: 42 mg

Pumpkin-Ginger Soup

MAKES 6 SERVINGS

Peeling is the most daunting part of preparing a pumpkin or squash. But when it's roasted first, peeling is a breeze.

- **3 pounds (1,360 g) fresh pumpkin or squash, or 2¼ cups (550 ml) mashed cooked pumpkin**
- **5 cups (1.25 L) water or vegetable broth**
- **1 large onion, chopped**
- **2 tablespoons (30 ml) light miso**
- **2 tablespoons (30 ml) peeled and grated fresh ginger**
- **1 tablespoon (15 ml) mild Indian curry paste**
- **½ red chile, seeded and diced, or ⅛ teaspoon (0.5 ml) cayenne** (optional)
- **½ teaspoon (2 ml) ground turmeric**
- **½ cup (125 ml) raw cashews**
- **¾ teaspoon (4 ml) salt** (optional)
- **Freshly ground black pepper**

Preheat the oven to 375 degrees F (190 degrees C). Line a baking sheet with parchment paper or a silicone baking mat.

Cut the pumpkin in half from the stem to the bottom. Scoop out and discard the seeds and membranes. Cut the halves into wedges.

Arrange the pumpkin in a single layer on the lined baking sheet. Bake for 30–40 minutes, until tender. Scoop out the flesh (discard the skin) and transfer it to a large soup pot. Add 4 cups (1 L) of the water and the onion, miso, ginger, curry paste, optional chile, and turmeric. Cook over medium heat, stirring occasionally, for 30 minutes. Transfer to a blender and process until smooth. Pour back into the soup pot.

Put the remaining 1 cup (250 ml) of water and the cashews in the blender and process until smooth and creamy. Pour into the soup and stir to combine. Cook over medium heat until warmed through, 2–3 minutes. Add the optional salt and season with pepper to taste. Serve hot.

Per serving
(1⅓ cups/325 ml):
calories: 92
protein: 3 g
fat: 5 g
carbohydrate: 10 g
dietary fiber: 2 g
calcium: 26 mg
sodium: 204 mg

Zesty Black Bean Soup

MAKES 7 CUPS
(1.75 L)

Beans and greens are the superstars of the Kick Diabetes diet. This thick and filling soup is loaded with flavor. Lime juice added just before serving contributes a bright note.

4 cups (1 L) water or vegetable broth

1 cup (250 ml) diced onion

1 cup (250 ml) diced celery

1 cup (250 ml) fresh or frozen corn or peeled and diced sweet potato

1 can (6 ounces/156 ml) tomato paste

3 cups (750 ml) unsalted cooked or canned black beans, drained and rinsed

2 cups (500 ml) chopped dark leafy greens (see Tip), packed

1 cup (250 ml) diced red bell pepper

2 cloves garlic, crushed

1 teaspoon (5 ml) dried oregano

1 teaspoon (5 ml) dried thyme

1 teaspoon (5 ml) salt

½ cup (125 ml) salsa (optional)

Freshly ground black pepper

2 tablespoons (30 ml) lime juice

For the greens, use bok choy, stemmed collard greens or kale, or fresh or frozen spinach.

Per 1 cup (250 ml):
calories: 175
protein: 10 g
fat: 1 g
carbohydrate: 35 g
dietary fiber: 10 g
calcium: 100 mg
sodium: 499 mg

Note: Analysis done with kale.

Put the water, onion, celery, and corn in a large soup pot and bring to a boil over medium-high heat. Decrease the heat to medium and cook, stirring occasionally, until the vegetables are almost tender, about 15 minutes. Add the tomato paste and stir until well combined. Add the beans, greens, bell pepper, garlic, oregano, thyme, and salt. Cook until the vegetables are tender, about 5 minutes. Add the optional salsa and stir to combine. Season with pepper to taste. Stir in the lime juice just before serving.

Hearty Split Pea, Lentil, and Barley Soup

MAKES 10 CUPS
(2.5 L)

Small legumes, such as split peas and lentils, are usually easier to digest than larger beans. The lentils and barley in this soup help stabilize blood sugar. For a flavor burst, garnish the soup with dehydrated sweet peppers and a drizzle of freshly squeezed lemon juice just before serving. Leftovers freeze well.

2 quarts (2 L) **water**

1 cup (250 ml) **dried red lentils**

1 cup (250 ml) **dried yellow split peas**

¾ cup (185 ml) **hulled or pot barley**

3 **carrots, sliced**

1 large **onion, chopped**

3 cloves **garlic, crushed**

2 teaspoons (10 ml) **dried basil**

2 teaspoons (10 ml) **salt**

1 **bay leaf**

Pinch **cayenne or ground cinnamon** (optional)

For a more intense garlic flavor, add the garlic during the last half hour of cooking.

Put the water, lentils, split peas, barley, carrots, onion, garlic, basil, salt, bay leaf, and optional cayenne in a large soup pot and bring to a boil over medium-high heat. Decrease the heat to medium-low, cover, and cook, stirring occasionally, until the barley is tender, about 1½ hours. Remove the bay leaf before serving. Serve hot.

VARIATION: Put 1 cup (250 ml) of stemmed and finely chopped kale, collard greens, Swiss chard, or spinach in each bowl before ladeling in the hot soup. The greens will wilt quickly and further increase the folate and fiber in the soup.

Per 1 cup (250 ml):
calories: 198
protein: 11 g
fat: 1 g
carbohydrate: 37 g
dietary fiber: 10 g
calcium: 37 mg
sodium: 489 mg

Curry in a Hurry Soup

MAKES 6 CUPS
(1.5 L)

Red lentils cook very quickly in this soup. If you prefer, use other types of lentils and simply increase the cooking time to about one hour. We recommend Patak's mild curry paste for the best flavor; it's generally available at major grocery stores and online.

4 cups (1 L) water or vegetable broth

1 onion, diced

1 cup (250 ml) dried red lentils

2 cups (500 ml) stemmed and chopped kale or spinach, packed

14 ounces (398 g) canned stewed or crushed tomatoes

1½ tablespoons (22 ml) mild Indian curry paste, plus more as needed

½ teaspoon (2 ml) salt

Freshly ground black pepper

Put the water, onion, and lentils in a large soup pot and bring to a boil over medium-high heat. Decrease the heat to medium-low, cover, and simmer until the lentils are tender, about 20 minutes. Add the kale, tomatoes, curry paste, and salt and stir to combine. Cook until the kale is tender, about 5 minutes. Season with pepper and additional curry paste to taste.

VARIATIONS: For even greater nutrition, increase the amount of kale or spinach or, along with the greens, add cooked cauliflower florets, jarred or canned tomatoes, diced bell peppers, or thinly sliced carrots. To further enhance the flavor, add chopped garlic, ginger, and/or 1 teaspoon (5 ml) ground turmeric along with the lentils.

Per 1 cup (250 ml):
calories: 161
protein: 10 g
fat: 2 g
carbohydrate: 27 g
dietary fiber: 7 g
calcium: 76 mg
sodium: 306 mg

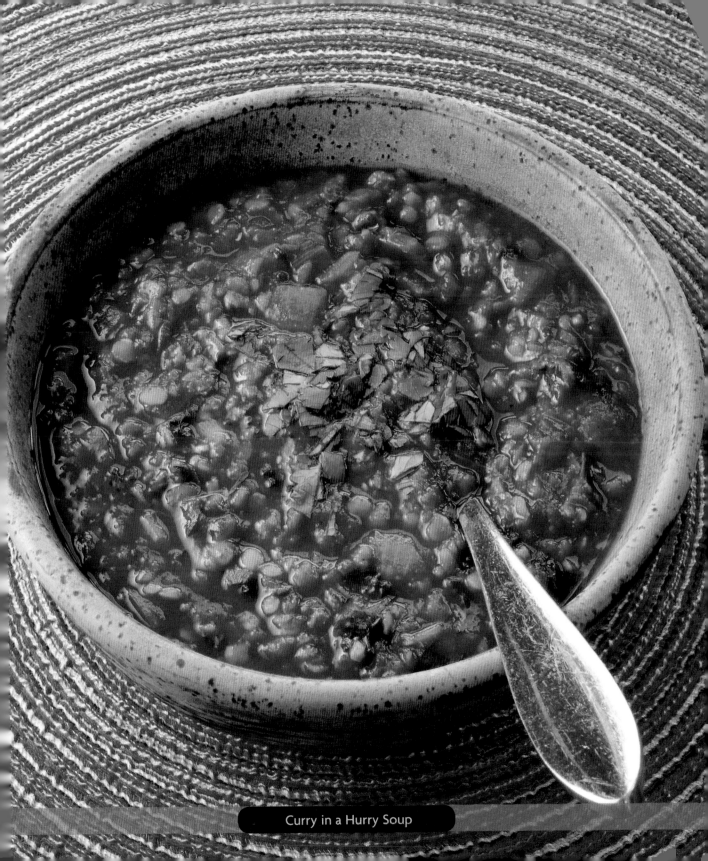

Curry in a Hurry Soup

Italian Minestrone

MAKES 10 CUPS
(2.50 L)

Almost any of the twenty types of beans that are commonly eaten will work in this recipe. Try cannellini beans, chickpeas, kidney beans, white beans, or whatever kind is your favorite.

4 cups (1 L) water or vegetable broth

2 cups (500 ml) chopped fresh or canned tomatoes, with juice

1 cup (250 ml) diced onion

1 cup (250 ml) diced carrot

1 cup (250 ml) diced celery

1 cup (250 ml) diced potato

2 tablespoons (30 ml) tomato paste

3 cloves garlic, crushed

1 teaspoon (5 ml) dried basil

1 teaspoon (5 ml) dried oregano

½ teaspoon (2 ml) whole celery seeds (optional)

½ teaspoon (2 ml) salt (optional)

1¾ cups (435 ml) cooked or canned beans (any kind)**, drained and rinsed**

1 cup (250 ml) sliced zucchini

1 cup (250 ml) cut green beans or yellow wax beans

Freshly ground black pepper

2 tablespoons (30 ml) chopped fresh parsley (optional)

Per 1 cup (250 ml):
calories: 94
protein: 5 g
fat: 0 g
carbohydrate: 19 g
dietary fiber: 6 g
calcium: 71 mg
sodium: 208 mg

Note: Analysis done with red kidney beans.

Put the water, tomatoes, onion, carrot, celery, potato, tomato paste, garlic, basil, oregano, optional celery seeds, and optional salt in a large soup pot and bring to a boil over medium-high heat. Decrease the heat to medium-low, cover, and simmer until the potato is almost cooked, about 15 minutes. Add the beans, zucchini, and green beans. Cover and cook until the vegetables are tender-crisp, 5–7 minutes. Season with pepper to taste. Serve hot, garnished with the optional parsley.

Full of Beans and Barley Soup

MAKES 7 CUPS
(1.75 L)

Beans and barley are the perfect combination for comfort and satiety, and for defeating diabetes. The least processed barley is hulled barley, followed by pot and then pearl. If possible, opt for hulled or pot barley.

4½ cups (1.125 L) **water or vegetable broth**

½ **onion, diced**

1 stalk celery, **diced**

1 carrot, **diced**

½ cup (125 ml) **hulled or pot barley**

1 teaspoon (5 ml) **dried basil, oregano, or savory**

1 teaspoon (5 ml) **dried rosemary**

1 teaspoon (5 ml) **dried thyme**

⅛ teaspoon (0.5 ml) **crushed red pepper flakes** (optional)

2 cups (500 ml) **stemmed and chopped dark leafy greens (see Tip), packed**

1 cup (250 ml) **chopped fresh tomatoes, or ¾ cup (185 ml) canned stewed tomatoes**

1 cup (250 ml) **cooked or canned red or white kidney beans, drained and rinsed**

3 cloves garlic, **crushed**

1 tablespoon (15 ml) **tamari**

¼ teaspoon (1 ml) **ground black pepper**

For the greens, use collard greens, kale, or spinach. Note that tender greens, such as spinach, will cook in about 3 minutes; tougher greens will cook in 5–10 minutes.

Put the water, onion, celery, carrot, barley, basil, rosemary, thyme, and optional red pepper flakes in a large soup pot and bring to a boil over medium-high heat. Decrease the heat to medium-low, cover, and cook, stirring occasionally, until the barley is tender, about 1 hour. If the mixture is dry, add a little more water.

Add the greens, tomatoes, beans, garlic, tamari, and pepper and stir to combine. Cover and cook, stirring occasionally, until heated through and the greens are tender, 3–10 minutes (see Tip). Serve hot.

VARIATIONS: For even more nutrition, include additional vegetables, such as sliced or chopped mushrooms, peeled and cubed winter squash, or diced turnips, when cooking the carrot and barley.

Per 1 cup (250 ml):
calories: 113
protein: 5 g
fat: 1 g
carbohydrate: 23 g
dietary fiber: 4 g
calcium: 115 mg
sodium: 169 mg

Note: Analysis done with kale.

Navy Bean and Mushroom Soup

MAKES 8 CUPS
(2 L)

Use different kinds of mushrooms to vary this delectable, creamy soup. Dried mushrooms soaked in water or vegetable broth can replace all or part of the fresh mushrooms.

½ cup (125 ml) **water or vegetable broth**

2 cups (500 ml) **sliced mushrooms**

2 **onions, chopped**

1 **carrot, diced**

3 **cloves garlic, crushed**

3 cups (750 ml) **cooked or canned navy beans, drained** (reserve liquid) **and rinsed**

3 cups (750 ml) **bean liquid, vegetable broth, or water**

2 tablespoons (30 ml) **tamari**

1 teaspoon (5 ml) **dried marjoram**

1 teaspoon (5 ml) **dried savory**

1 teaspoon (5 ml) **dried thyme**

1 teaspoon (5 ml) **ground turmeric**

½ teaspoon (2 ml) **salt**

Freshly ground black pepper

Put the water, mushrooms, onions, carrot, and garlic in a large soup pot and bring to a boil over medium-high heat. Decrease the heat to medium-low, cover, and cook for 10 minutes.

Put 1½ cups (375 ml) of the beans and 1½ cups (375 ml) of the bean liquid in a blender and process until smooth. Pour into the soup pot. Add the remaining 1½ cups (375 ml) of the beans, the remaining 1½ cups (375 ml) of the bean liquid, and the tamari, marjoram, savory, thyme, turmeric, and salt. Season with pepper to taste. Cover and simmer over low heat, stirring occasionally, until hot, about 10 minutes.

Per 1 cup (250 ml):
calories: 103
protein: 6 g
fat: 1 g
carbohydrate: 19 g
dietary fiber: 7 g
calcium: 55 mg
sodium: 345 mg

Black-Eyed Pea and Eggplant Soup

This soup is easy to prepare, and the unexpected combination of herbs and spices makes it a real treat.

MAKES 8 CUPS (2 L)

3 cups (750 ml) water or vegetable broth

1 eggplant

1 onion, chopped

1 small green bell pepper, diced

2½ cups (625 ml) cooked or canned black-eyed peas, drained and rinsed

2 cups (500 ml) pureed fresh or canned tomatoes

1 teaspoon (5 ml) dried basil

1 teaspoon (5 ml) dried thyme

1 teaspoon (5 ml) ground nutmeg

½ teaspoon (2 ml) salt

Put ½ cup (125 ml) of the water and the eggplant, onion, and bell pepper in a large soup pot. Cover and cook over medium-low heat, stirring occasionally, until the vegetables are soft, about 10 minutes. Add the remaining 2½ cups (625 ml) of the water and the black-eyed peas, tomatoes, basil, thyme, nutmeg, and salt and stir to combine. Cook, stirring frequently, for 15 minutes. Remove from the heat, cover, and let rest for 10 minutes before serving to allow the flavors to blend. Serve hot.

Per 1 cup (250 ml):
calories: 107
protein: 6 g
fat: 1 g
carbohydrate: 21 g
dietary fiber: 7 g
calcium: 51 mg
sodium: 233 mg

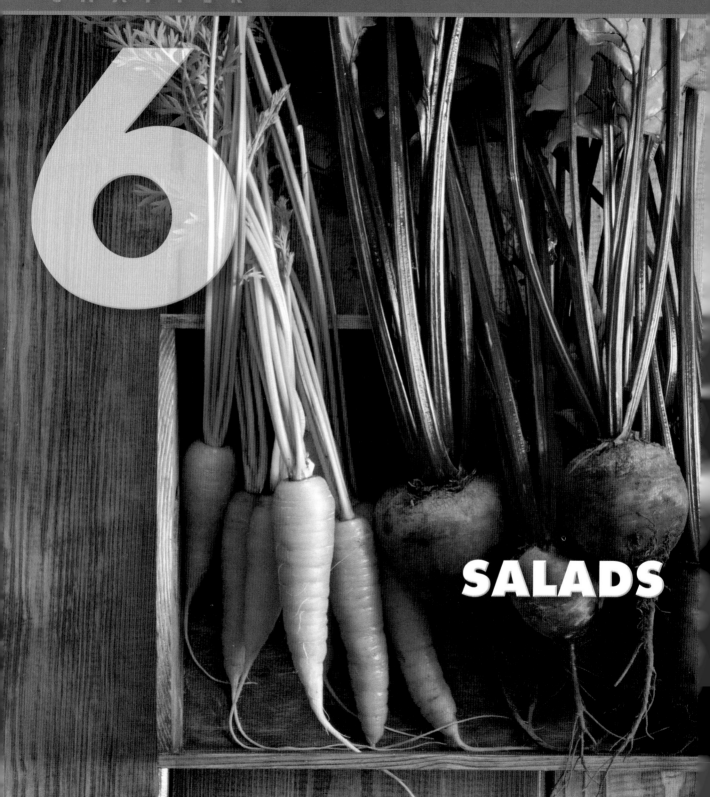

6

SALADS

Five-Day Salad

MAKES 10 CUPS
(2.5 L)

I f you make this calcium-rich salad once or twice a week, you'll have plenty on hand when you walk in the door hungry. Do the chopping while listening to your favorite music, or make it a shared activity with a family member or friend.

- **3 cups (750 ml) stemmed and very thinly sliced kale or collard greens, packed**
- **3 cups (750 ml) bite-size pieces romaine lettuce, lightly packed**
- **3 cups (750 ml) thinly sliced napa cabbage**
- **1 cup (250 ml) very thinly sliced or finely chopped red cabbage**

Put the kale, lettuce, napa cabbage, and red cabbage in a large bowl and toss to combine.

VARIATIONS: For a heartier salad, add additional veggies (such as grated carrot, chopped bell pepper, whole or halved cherry tomatoes, and other vegetables or fruits) just before serving. Include well-cooked grains and beans to make it a full meal.

Stored in a sealed container in the refrigerator, the salad will keep for 5 days. Toss just the amount you need with your favorite salad dressing right before serving.

INSTANT SALAD

For an almost-instant salad, shop for triple-washed greens, cherry tomatoes, and grated carrots. Toss in some cooked beans and grains, and your colorful, nutritious salad will come together in minutes.

Per 2 cups (500 ml):
calories: 46
protein: 3 g
fat: 0.5 g
carbohydrate: 9 g
dietary fiber: 3 g
calcium: 126 mg
sodium: 35 mg

Classic Broccoli Salad

MAKES 3½ CUPS
(875 ML),
3 SERVINGS

Nutrient-packed broccoli is brimming with vitamins A and C, calcium, and folic acid. It also has the perfect balance of soluble and insoluble fiber. As a member of the cruciferous family, broccoli boasts an abundance of protective phytochemicals and contains an enzyme that helps convert its phytochemicals to more active, cancer-fighting forms.

3 cups (750 ml) small broccoli florets

Peeled and grated broccoli stem (optional)

1 carrot, grated

¼ small red onion, finely diced (optional)

⅞ cup (220 ml) Orange-Ginger Dressing (page 106)**, or ½ cup** (125 ml) **Lemon-Tahini Dressing** (page 104)

¼ cup (60 ml) dried currants or raisins, plus more for garnish

2 tablespoons (30 ml) raw sunflower seeds, pumpkin seeds, or chopped almonds, plus more for garnish

Steam the broccoli florets and optional stem until tender-crisp, 2–3 minutes. Transfer to a medium bowl and add the carrot and optional onion. Add the dressing and stir until the vegetables are evenly coated. Add the currants and sunflower seeds and toss until evenly distributed. Garnish with additional currants and sunflower seeds. Serve immediately.

Per serving:

calories: 187

protein: 6 g

fat: 5 g

carbohydrate: 36 g

dietary fiber: 6 g

calcium: 88 mg

sodium: 314 mg

Green Potato Salad with Dill

MAKES 5 CUPS
(1.25 L)

Avocado makes this unique potato salad naturally creamy, and fresh dill imparts a captivating flavor. Use more or less lemon juice, lime juice, or apple cider vinegar to suit your taste.

5 cups (1.25 L) diced potatoes

1 large avocado

3 tablespoons (45 ml) apple cider vinegar

3 tablespoons (45 ml) chopped fresh dill, or 1 tablespoon (15 ml) dried dill weed

2 tablespoons (30 ml) lemon or lime juice

1½ tablespoons (22 ml) Dijon mustard

½ teaspoon (2 ml) ground black pepper

2 dill pickles, diced

1½ stalks celery, diced

¼ teaspoon (1 ml) salt (optional)

Put the potatoes in a medium saucepan, cover with water, and bring to a boil over medium-high heat. Decrease the heat to medium, cover, and cook until the potatoes are just tender, about 15 minutes. Drain and let cool.

Scoop the avocado flesh into a large bowl and mash with a fork. Add the vinegar, dill, lemon juice, mustard, and pepper and stir until evenly distributed. Add the pickles, celery, and optional salt and stir until well combined. Add the potatoes and gently stir until evenly coated. Cover tightly and refrigerate for 1–2 hours before serving. Serve well chilled.

Per 1 cup (250 ml):
calories: 182
protein: 4 g
fat: 6 g
carbohydrate: 31 g
dietary fiber: 6 g
calcium: 43 mg
sodium: 316 mg

Kale Salad with Orange-Ginger Dressing

MAKES 3½ CUPS
(875 ML),
3 SERVINGS

f you don't know what to do with kale, here's a delicious way to prepare this famously nutritious green. It's best cut matchstick thin. To tenderize the kale further, you can massage it for about five minutes or marinate it in the dressing for up to one day in advance, before you add the remaining ingredients.

6 cups (1.5 L) **stemmed and thinly sliced kale, packed**

1 cup (250 ml) **thinly sliced red cabbage**

1 **carrot, grated or julienned**

½ **red bell pepper, thinly sliced**

2 tablespoons (30 ml) **chopped fresh parsley or cilantro**

2 tablespoons (30 ml) **chopped fresh mint** (optional)

⅞ **cup** (220 ml) **Orange-Ginger Dressing** (page 106)

¼ **cup** (60 ml) **raw sunflower, sesame, or chia seeds** (optional)

Put the kale, cabbage, carrot, bell pepper, parsley, and optional mint in a large bowl and toss to combine. Add the dressing and toss until evenly distributed. Let marinate for at least 20 minutes. Sprinkle with the optional sunflower seeds just before serving.

Per serving:
calories: 261
protein: 11 g
fat: 8 g
carbohydrate: 45 g
dietary fiber: 9 g
calcium: 310 mg
sodium: 376 mg

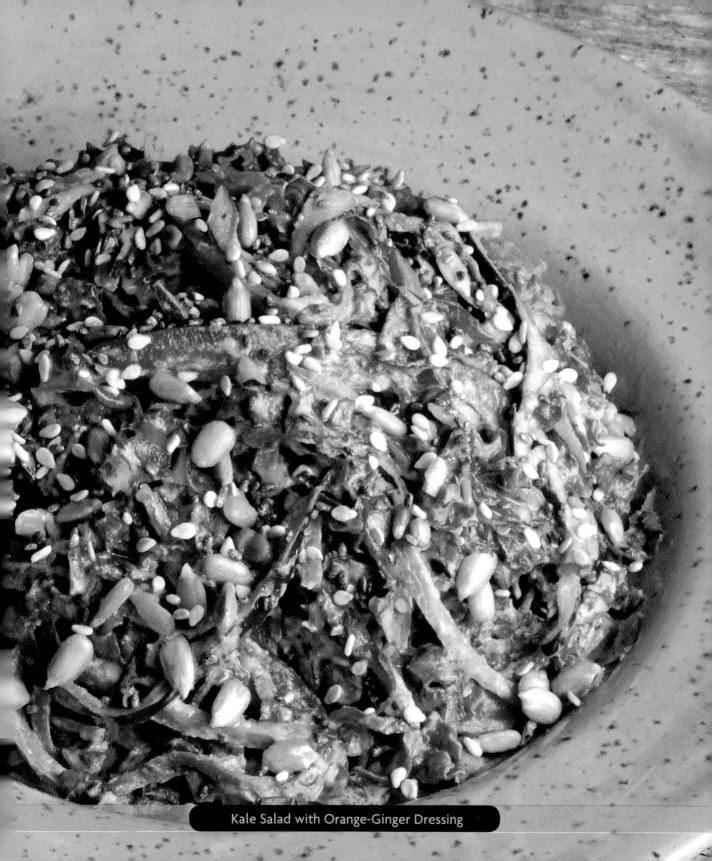

Kale Salad with Orange-Ginger Dressing

Cabbage Carrot Slaw

MAKES 5½ CUPS
(1.38 L),
4 SERVINGS

To speed the process of making this crunchy salad, use a food processor to slice the cabbage, grate the carrots, and chop the parsley.

6 cups (1.5 L) shredded savoy or green cabbage

1⅔ cups (415 ml) Cashew Mayonnaise (page 109)

3 medium carrots, grated, or 1 cup (250 ml) grated carrots, packed

½ cup (125 ml) chopped fresh parsley, lightly packed

⅓ cup (85 ml) roasted sunflower seeds

2 tablespoons (30 ml) spicy brown mustard

2 tablespoons (30 ml) whole caraway seeds

1 teaspoon (5 ml) whole celery seeds

¼ teaspoon (1 ml) salt

Put all the ingredients in a large bowl and toss until well combined.

Per serving:
calories: 338
protein: 12 g
fat: 22 g
carbohydrate: 30 g
dietary fiber: 8 g
calcium: 127 mg
sodium: 457 mg

Raw Vegetable Platter

olorful vegetables, artfully cut and attractively arranged on a platter, have much to offer:

- an appealing way to present veggies at mealtimes
- a healthy, low-calorie snack while watching TV
- an artistic accompaniment to festive meals
- a great way to get vitamins, phytochemicals, antioxidants, and fiber

A beautiful platter also encourages family members to eat their veggies when they come home from school or work. If you've never eaten raw corn on the cob (without butter), give it a try—it's wonderful! Here's a list of items you can serve on a raw-vegetable platter, straight up or with one of the dips on pages 111–115:

- **Asparagus tips**
- **Broccoli florets**
- **Carrot sticks**
- **Cauliflower florets**
- **Celery sticks**
- **Cherry tomatoes**
- **Cucumber rounds**
- **Green onions**
- **Jicama sticks**
- **Parsnip rounds or sticks**
- **Radishes, whole, halved, or sliced**
- **Red, yellow, and/or green bell pepper strips**
- **Snow peas**
- **Sugar snap peas**
- **Sweet potato strips** (dipped in water with a little lemon juice to prevent browning)
- **Turnip sticks**
- **Yam strips**
- **Zucchini rounds or sticks**

Quinoa-Broccoli Salad with Lime Dressing

MAKES 3½ CUPS
(875 ML)

Quinoa is rightfully known as a supergrain because of its high protein content and outstanding nutritional profile. The magnesium and potassium content is especially helpful for people with diabetes. It's also quick to cook!

1½ cups (375 ml) **cooked quinoa** (see page 56)

1 cup (250 ml) **small broccoli florets or chopped broccolini, lightly steamed**

1 cup (250 ml) **cooked green peas**

¼ cup (60 ml) **diced red or orange bell pepper**

¼ cup (60 ml) **diced cucumber** (optional)

2 tablespoons (30 ml) **finely chopped fresh parsley or cilantro**

3 tablespoons (45 ml) **lime or lemon juice**

1 tablespoon (15 ml) **tamari, or ¼ teaspoon (1 ml) salt**

Pinch **ground black pepper or cayenne**

3 tablespoons (45 ml) **raw or roasted pumpkin seeds**

Put the quinoa, broccoli, peas, bell pepper, optional cucumber, and parsley in a medium bowl and stir to combine. Add the lime juice, tamari, and pepper and toss gently with a fork until evenly distributed. Sprinkle with the pumpkin seeds just before serving. Serve warm or cold.

If time permits, cover and refrigerate for 1–3 hours before serving to let the flavors blend.

Per one-third recipe:
calories: 231
protein: 11 g
fat: 7 g
carbohydrate: 33 g
dietary fiber: 6 g
calcium: 47 mg
sodium: 391 mg

Ruby Red Salad

MAKES 6 CUPS
(1.5 L)

This jewel-like salad is excellent tossed with Orange-Ginger Dressing (page 106), Lemon-Tahini Dressing (page 104), or Liquid Gold Dressing with Zucchini and Hemp Seeds (page 108). Alternatively, offer several dressings at the table and let everyone choose their own.

3 cups (750 ml) **grated carrots**

2 cups (500 ml) **grated beets**

1 cup (250 ml) **chopped fresh parsley, lightly packed**

½ **cup** (125 ml) **coarsely chopped walnuts**

½ **cup** (125 ml) **pomegranate seeds**

2 tablespoons (30 ml) **thinly sliced fresh chives** (optional)

Salad dressing of choice (see pages 104–109)

½ **teaspoon** (2 ml) **salt** (optional)

Freshly ground black pepper

Put the carrots, beets, parsley, walnuts, pomegranate seeds, and optional chives in a large bowl. Add salad dressing to taste and stir until the vegetables are evenly coated. Add the optional salt and season with pepper to taste. Serve immediately.

VARIATION: Add 1 or 2 diced red apples.

To remove seeds from a pomegranate, roll the fruit first to loosen the seeds. Then cut the pomegranate skin to halve or quarter the fruit and remove seeds with a spoon.

Per 1 cup (250 ml):
calories: 111
protein: 3 g
fat: 7 g
carbohydrate: 12 g
dietary fiber: 3 g
calcium: 47 mg
sodium: 65 mg

Note: Analysis doesn't include salad dressing.

Cauliflower and Basmati Rice Salad

MAKES 4 CUPS
(1 L)

Raisins, curry paste (such as Patak's mild curry paste), cauliflower florets, and brown basmati rice join forces in this delicious and colorful salad.

3 cups (750 ml) small cauliflower florets

1 cup (250 ml) cooked brown basmati rice or brown rice

¾ cup (185 ml) diced red bell pepper

¾ cup (185 ml) chopped fresh parsley or cilantro, lightly packed

¼ cup (60 ml) raisins, soaked in hot water for 30 minutes and drained

2 tablespoons (30 ml) mild Indian curry paste

3 tablespoons (45 ml) lemon or lime juice

Steam the cauliflower for 5 minutes. Transfer to a medium bowl and add the rice, bell pepper, parsley, and raisins.

Put the curry paste In a small bowl. Add the lemon juice and stir until well combined. Add to the rice mixture and gently stir with a fork until evenly distributed. Serve immediately.

VARIATIONS: Stir in ¼ teaspoon (1 ml) ground turmeric and 1 teaspoon (5 ml) ground coriander along with the curry paste, and/or replace one-third of the parsley with chopped fresh mint or basil. To turn this salad into a main dish, add 1½ cups (375 ml) cooked or canned lentils or mung beans.

Per 1 cup (250 ml):
calories: 130
protein: 4 g
fat: 3 g
carbohydrate: 28 g
dietary fiber: 5 g
calcium: 41 mg
sodium: 130 mg

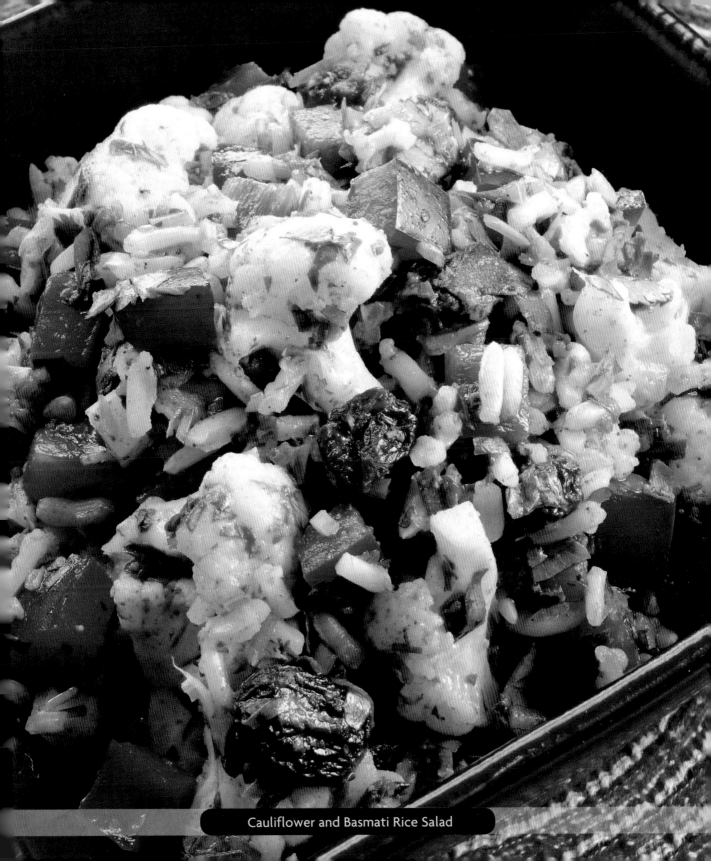

Cauliflower and Basmati Rice Salad

Full-Meal Salad

MAKES 2–3 SERVINGS

Choose a mix from the following categories for an abundant and filling salad and a feast of protective phytochemicals. Whenever possible, choose organic produce.

Green and Leafy Vegetables. Use a total of about 8 cups (2 L). Here is a suggested combination:

- 4 cups (1 L) mixed salad greens, lightly packed
- 2 cups (500 ml) stemmed and very thinly sliced kale, packed
- 2 cups (500 ml) chopped radicchio or thinly sliced red or purple cabbage

Colorful Vegetables. Cover the rainbow in your selection of veggies with 1 cup (250 ml) from each of the five color families below:

GREEN
- Asparagus, sliced diagonally (raw or steamed)
- Avocado, sliced or cubed
- Broccolini or broccoli florets and stems, sliced diagonally
- Cucumber, sliced
- Snow peas or sugar snap peas
- Sprouts (pea, sunflower, or other)
- Zucchini or celery, sliced

YELLOW-ORANGE
- Golden cauliflower, cut into small florets
- Yellow beets, grated or cooked (baked, steamed, or boiled) and cubed
- Yellow or orange bell pepper, cut into wide strips
- Yellow or orange carrots, sliced or grated

PINK-RED
- Beets (steamed, boiled, or raw), cubed or grated
- Red bell pepper, cut into wide strips
- Red onion, thinly sliced
- Tomatoes (cherry, grape, or other)
- Watermelon radish, cut into small cubes or strips

PURPLE-BLUE
- Blueberries, blackberries, or halved black grapes
- Purple bell pepper, cut into wide strips
- Purple carrots, sliced or grated
- Purple cauliflower, cut into small florets

WHITE
- Cauliflower, cut into small florets
- Kohlrabi or jicama, cut into thin strips
- Salad turnips, sliced
- Sweet onion, thinly sliced

Herbs. For a flavor boost, mix in ½ cup (125 ml) chopped fresh basil, dill, parsley, or other fresh herbs.

Plant-Protein Superstars. Choose at least 1 or 2 of these high-protein foods:
- 6–8 ounces (170–225 g) smoked tofu, cubed
- 6–8 ounces (170–225 g) tofu, cubed and baked or sautéed with tamari, turmeric, herbs, and spices
- 6–8 ounces (170–225 g) tempeh, baked or steamed, and cubed
- 1–2 cups (250–500 ml) chickpeas, other beans, or lentils
- ¼ cup (60 ml) peanuts, pumpkin seeds, sunflower seeds, or other nuts or seeds
- 4–8 falafels or other veggie balls

Starches. To make the meal even more satisfying, include 1 cup (250 ml) or more of the following:
- Cooked basmati rice, brown rice, Kamut berries, quinoa, spelt berries, or wild rice
- Corn, raw or cooked
- Sweet potato, butternut squash, other winter squash, or purple or white potato, steamed and cubed

Nut- or Seed-Based Dressing. Choose from the dressings on pages 104–109.

Put the green and leafy vegetables in a large bowl. Top with the colorful vegetables and herbs and stir until well combined. If the entire salad will be served at once, add the plant protein and starches. If you're going to save some for another day, store the protein superstars and starches (and avocado, if using) separately so they can be added fresh just before serving. Mix in the salad dressing just before serving or serve it on the side.

Mango and Black Bean Salad

MAKES 3 CUPS
(750 ML)

njoy this salad on its own, or serve it on a bed of cooked or raw greens (or have the greens on the side).

1 mango, diced

1 small red bell pepper, diced

1 cup (250 ml) cooked or canned black beans, drained and rinsed

2 tablespoons (30 ml) lime juice

1 tablespoon (15 ml) chopped fresh parsley or cilantro

¼ teaspoon (1 ml) salt

¼ teaspoon (1 ml) ground black pepper

Diced avocado (optional)

Put the mango, bell pepper, beans, lime juice, parsley, salt, and pepper in a medium bowl and stir to combine. Let stand for 10 minutes before serving to allow the flavors to blend. Top with avocado if desired.

Per 1 cup (250 ml):
calories: 123
protein: 6 g
fat: 1 g
carbohydrate: 26 g
dietary fiber: 6 g
calcium: 26 mg
sodium: 200 mg

Sun-Dried Tomato, Bean, and Barley Salad

Sun-dried tomatoes add tang and color to this hearty salad. Arugula has a strong flavor that many people adore, but if you don't care for it, try baby kale, bok choy, spinach, or a mix of other greens instead.

MAKES 6 CUPS
(1.5 L)

½ cup (125 ml) **sun-dried tomatoes**

½ cup (125 ml) **boiling water**

2 cups (500 ml) **cooked barley** (any kind)**, cooled and rinsed**

2 cups (500 ml) **finely chopped arugula or other greens, lightly packed**

1 cup (250 ml) **cooked or canned black, red, or adzuki beans, drained and rinsed**

1 fresh tomato, diced, or 1 cup (250 ml) **halved cherry tomatoes**

½ cup (125 ml) **chopped fresh basil or parsley, lightly packed**

2 cloves garlic, crushed

¼ cup (60 ml) **sunflower or pumpkin seeds**

3 tablespoons (45 ml) **lemon juice**

3 tablespoons (45 ml) **balsamic vinegar**

2 teaspoons (10 ml) **tamari**

⅛ teaspoon (0.5 ml) **ground black pepper**

Put the sun-dried tomatoes in a small heatproof bowl. Add the boiling water and let the tomatoes soak until soft, about 20 minutes. Drain, chop, and transfer to a medium bowl. Add the barley, arugula, beans, fresh tomato, basil, and garlic and stir to combine. Add the sunflower seeds, lemon juice, vinegar, tamari, and pepper and gently toss with a fork until well distributed. Stored in a sealed container in the refrigerator, the salad will keep for 3 days.

Per 1 cup (250 ml):
calories: 189
protein: 8 g
fat: 4 g
carbohydrate: 34 g
dietary fiber: 9 g
calcium: 54 mg
sodium: 222 mg

Kamut, Kale, Tomato, and Avocado Salad

MAKES 6 CUPS
(1.5 L)

Kamut is an ancient grain that's closely related to wheat. It has a sweet taste and a soft, chewy texture that works well in this nutritious full-meal salad. Some people with a sensitivity to common wheat find that they can tolerate Kamut and spelt (which also works well in this recipe). For people who need to avoid gluten entirely, wild rice makes an excellent stand-in for the Kamut.

2 cups (500 ml) stemmed and finely chopped kale, packed

1½ cups (375 ml) cooked Kamut or spelt berries

1½ cups (375 ml) cooked or canned kidney beans, drained and rinsed

1 cup (250 ml) diced cucumber

1 cup (250 ml) halved cherry tomatoes, or 1 tomato, diced

3 tablespoons (45 ml) chopped fresh basil or dill, or 1 cup (250 ml) chopped fresh parsley, lightly packed

2 cloves garlic, crushed

3 tablespoons (45 ml) lemon juice

3 tablespoons (45 ml) balsamic vinegar

2 teaspoons (10 ml) tamari

1 avocado, diced or sliced

If you don't have fresh herbs on hand, use dried. For each tablespoon (15 ml) of fresh herbs, use 1 teaspoon (5 ml) dried.

Put the kale, Kamut, beans, cucumber, tomatoes, basil, and garlic in a large bowl and stir to combine. Add the lemon juice, vinegar, and tamari and stir until evenly distributed. Gently stir in the avocado or arrange it on top. Serve immediately.

Per 1 cup (250 ml):
calories: 190
protein: 8 g
fat: 5 g
carbohydrate: 31 g
dietary fiber: 9 g
calcium: 77 mg
sodium: 129 mg

Sweet Potato and Chickpea Salad

his is a dish you'll want to make again and again. It can be served at room temperature over a bed of arugula or other salad greens or over steamed dark leafy greens.

MAKES 4 CUPS (1 L)

1 large sweet potato, peeled if desired and cubed

1¾ cups (435 ml) cooked or canned chickpeas, drained (save the liquid) and rinsed

1 red bell pepper, diced

⅓ cup (85 ml) golden or dark raisins

2 tablespoons (30 ml) nutritional yeast flakes

2 tablespoons (30 ml) tahini

2 tablespoons (30 ml) water or chickpea liquid

2 tablespoons (30 ml) fortified unsweetened soy milk or other nondairy milk

1 tablespoon (15 ml) Dijon mustard

1 tablespoon (15 ml) apple cider vinegar

2 teaspoons (10 ml) prepared horseradish

1½ teaspoons (7 ml) peeled and grated fresh ginger, or ⅛ teaspoon (0.5 ml) ground ginger

½ teaspoon (2 ml) ground turmeric

¼ teaspoon (1 ml) salt

¼ teaspoon (1 ml) ground black pepper

3 tablespoons (45 ml) chopped fresh cilantro or parsley, plus more for garnish

Steam the sweet potato until soft but still firm enough to keep its shape, 5–10 minutes. Drain and rinse under cold water to quickly cool.

Put the chickpeas in a medium bowl and coarsely mash, leaving some beans intact. Add the sweet potato, bell pepper, and raisins and stir to combine.

Put the nutritional yeast, tahini, water, milk, mustard, vinegar, horseradish, ginger, turmeric, salt, and pepper in a small glass jar. Seal the jar tightly and shake until well combined. Pour over the sweet potato mixture, add the cilantro, and gently stir until evenly distributed. Garnish with additional cilantro before serving.

Per 1 cup (250 ml):
calories: 271
protein: 10 g
fat: 6 g
carbohydrate: 46 g
dietary fiber: 9 g
calcium: 75 mg
sodium: 276 mg

Multicolor Bean and Vegetable Salad

MAKES 6 CUPS
(1.5 L)

Make your own salad with the following guide for a meal you're sure to enjoy. Serve it over a bed of torn or chopped fresh salad greens.

MARINADE

2 tablespoons (30 ml) **white balsamic vinegar, apple cider vinegar, or lemon juice**

1 tablespoon (15 ml) **fresh dill, or 1 teaspoon (5 ml) dried dill weed**

1 teaspoon (5 ml) **minced garlic or garlic powder**

1 teaspoon (5 ml) **Dijon mustard**

1½ teaspoons (7 ml) **light miso**

Freshly ground black pepper

BEANS

3 cups (750 ml) **cooked or canned beans** (one type or a combination of several), **drained and rinsed**

VEGETABLES

3 cups (750 ml) **of two or more of the following vegetables, or use whatever vegetables you have on hand:**

- Asparagus, sliced diagonally and steamed until tender-crisp
- Bell peppers, diced
- Broccoli florets
- Cauliflower florets
- Celery, diced
- Cherry tomatoes, halved
- Corn, fresh or frozen and thawed
- Green beans, cut into 2-inch lengths and steamed until tender-crisp
- Napa cabbage, sliced
- Snow peas, whole or sliced diagonally
- Zucchini, sliced or diced

CONDIMENTS (OPTIONAL)

- Olives, whole or sliced
- Pickled artichoke hearts
- Pickles, sliced or diced

To make the marinade, put the vinegar, dill, garlic, and mustard in a small jar. Add the miso and press it with a spoon to help disperse it. Seal tightly and shake until well combined. Season with pepper to taste.

Put the beans in a large bowl. Add the marinade and stir to coat the beans. Cover and refrigerate for at least 6 hours, stirring occasionally. Mix in the vegetables and optional condiments of your choice just before serving.

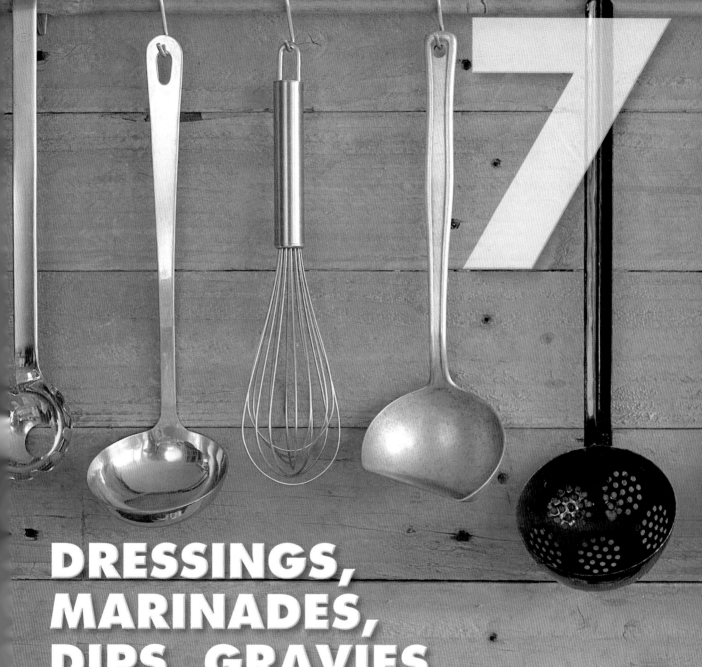

7

DRESSINGS, MARINADES, DIPS, GRAVIES, AND SAUCES

Lemon-Tahini Dressing

MAKES 1⅓ CUPS
(325 ML)

Tahini can be used to flavor sauces and soups or to make salad dressings creamy. If the oil rises to the top, just give it a good stir before using. This dressing can also be used as a sauce for steamed broccoli and other vegetables, baked potatoes, or beans. Freshly squeezed lemon or lime juice provides better flavor than bottled, along with more vitamin C and no sulfites.

½ cup (125 ml) **water**

⅓ cup (85 ml) **tahini**

⅓ cup (85 ml) **lemon or lime juice**

1 tablespoon (15 ml) **tamari**

2 cloves garlic, crushed

Pinch cayenne (optional)

Put the water, tahini, lemon juice, tamari, garlic, and optional cayenne in a blender and process until smooth, about 30 seconds. Stored in a sealed container in the refrigerator, the dressing will keep for 3 weeks.

Use 2 tablespoons (30 ml) of dressing for a side salad and ¼ cup (60 ml) for a main-dish salad.

Per ¼ cup (60 ml):
calories: 98
protein: 3 g
fat: 8 g
carbohydrate: 5 g
dietary fiber: 1.5 g
calcium: 69 mg
sodium: 211 mg

Limey Avocado Dip or Dressing

ake this dip right before you're ready to use it so it will retain its attractive color. The addition of water will make it thin enough to use as a dressing.

MAKES ¾ CUP
(185 ML)

1 avocado

2 tablespoons (30 ml) lime juice

1 tablespoon (15 ml) nutritional yeast flakes

½ teaspoon (2 ml) chili powder

½ teaspoon (2 ml) garlic powder

½ teaspoon (2 ml) onion powder

¼ teaspoon (1 ml) salt, or 1 teaspoon (5 ml) tamari

Pinch ground black pepper

¼ cup (60 ml) water or vegetable broth, as needed (optional)

Scoop the avocado flesh into a small bowl and mash it with a fork until smooth. Alternatively, mash it using an immersion blender for a smoother mixture. Stir in the lime juice, nutritional yeast, chili powder, garlic powder, onion powder, salt, and pepper. For a dressing, add just enough of the optional water to achieve the desired consistency.

Per 2 tablespoons
(30 ml):
calories: 59
protein: 1 g
fat: 5 g
carbohydrate: 4 g
dietary fiber: 2 g
calcium: 6 mg
sodium: 105 mg

Hummus and Lime Dressing

MAKES 1 CUP
(250 ML)

Per ¼ cup (60 ml):
calories: 58
protein: 2 g
fat: 3 g
carbohydrate: 7 g
dietary fiber: 1 g
calcium: 17 mg
sodium: 75 mg

This versatile dressing is a snap to make, especially if you have ready-made hummus on hand. Use one of the varieties of Heart-warming Hummus (page 113) or try your favorite flavor of store-bought hummus.

⅓ cup (85 ml) water

½ cup (125 ml) hummus

2 tablespoons (30 ml) lime or lemon juice

1 teaspoon (5 ml) ground turmeric or dried dill weed

Put the water in a blender. Add the hummus, lime juice, and turmeric and process until smooth.

Orange-Ginger Dressing

MAKES ⅞ CUP
(220 ML)

Per 2 tablespoons
(30 ml):
calories: 74
protein: 2 g
fat: 4 g
carbohydrate: 9 g
dietary fiber: 2 g
calcium: 32 mg
sodium: 122 mg

Ginger lovers, this dressing is for you! Increase the amount of ginger if you want the flavor to be even more pronounced.

1 orange, peeled and seeded

1½ tablespoons (22 ml) tahini

2 pitted soft dates

1 tablespoon (15 ml) peeled and grated fresh ginger

1½ teaspoons (7 ml) light miso

1 tablespoon (15 ml) apple cider vinegar

1½ teaspoons (7 ml) tamari

Pinch cayenne or ground black pepper

Put the orange, tahini, dates, ginger, and miso in a blender and process until well combined. Add the vinegar, tamari, and cayenne and process until smooth.

Creamy Hemp Dressing

MAKES 2 CUPS (500 ML)

This creamy dressing is rich in omega-3 fatty acids yet is low in fat and calories. Just three tablespoons (45 ml) of hemp seeds provide 10 grams of high-quality protein, 3 grams of omega-3 fatty acids, and an impressive array of minerals, including iron, zinc, potassium, and magnesium.

1 cup (250 ml) **water**

¾ cup (185 ml) **hemp seeds**

⅓ cup (85 ml) **lemon juice or white balsamic vinegar**

1 tablespoon (15 ml) **light miso**

3 small pitted dates, or 1 large pitted date

1 tablespoon (15 ml) **stone-ground or Dijon mustard**

1 clove garlic, crushed

Put all the ingredients in a blender and process until smooth. Stored in a sealed container in the refrigerator, the dressing will keep for 2 weeks.

VARIATION: To boost intake of B vitamins, add ¼ cup (60 ml) nutritional yeast flakes before blending. For a reliable source of vitamin B_{12}, use Red Star Vegetarian Support Formula nutritional yeast or another brand that shows vitamin B_{12} on the label.

Per ¼ cup (60 ml):
calories: 102
protein: 6 g
fat: 7 g
carbohydrate: 5 g
dietary fiber: 1 g
calcium: 10 mg
sodium: 113 mg

Liquid Gold Dressing with Zucchini and Hemp Seeds

MAKES 2 CUPS
(500 ML)

This dressing supplies omega-3 fatty acids and is packed with B vitamins. When it's made with nutritional yeast that's grown on a B_{12}-enriched medium, it also delivers vitamin B_{12}. The zucchini creates a dressing that's relatively low in fat but still has body. If you opt not to peel the zucchini, the dressing will have a green tinge.

2 cups (500 ml) zucchini, peeled and chopped

¾ cup (185 ml) hemp seeds

½ cup (125 ml) lemon juice, lime juice, or apple cider vinegar

½ cup (125 ml) nutritional yeast flakes

¼ cup (60 ml) tamari

4 teaspoons (20 ml) ground flaxseeds

1 teaspoon (5 ml) Dijon mustard

1 teaspoon (5 ml) ground cumin

1 teaspoon (5 ml) ground turmeric

2 cloves garlic, crushed

Put all the ingredients in a blender and process until smooth. Stored in a sealed container in the refrigerator, the dressing will keep for 4 days.

If the dressing gets too thick in the fridge, thin it with a small amount of water, lemon juice, or lime juice before serving.

Per 2 tablespoons
(30 ml):
calories: 61
protein: 4 g
fat: 4 g
carbohydrate: 4 g
dietary fiber: 1 g
calcium: 12 mg
sodium: 261 mg

Cashew Mayonnaise

This delicious, creamy dressing can take the place of traditional mayonnaise in any recipe. Use it sparingly, though, as it is quite rich.

MAKES 1⅔ CUPS (415 ML)

1 cup (250 ml) raw cashews, soaked in water for 1–4 hours, drained, and rinsed

¼ cup (60 ml) lemon juice

¼ cup (60 ml) water, plus more as needed

2 tablespoons (30 ml) apple cider vinegar

1 teaspoon (5 ml) spicy brown mustard

1 clove garlic, crushed

¼ teaspoon (1 ml) salt

Put all the ingredients in a blender and process until smooth and creamy. If the mixture is too thick, add a little more water, 1 teaspoon (5 ml) at a time, until the desired consistency is achieved. Stored in a sealed container in the refrigerator, the mayonnaise will keep for 1 week.

Per 2 tablespoons (30 ml):
calories: 56
protein: 2 g
fat: 4 g
carbohydrate: 4 g
dietary fiber: 0 g
calcium: 5 mg
sodium: 50 mg

Tofu or Tempeh Marinade

MAKES ⅞ CUP
(220 ML)

Tofu and tempeh are like blank canvases. Their ability to readily absorb flavors makes them incredibly versatile foods that are perfect for marinating. This marinade can also be used as a stir-fry sauce or to baste grilled vegetables, and it's delicious drizzled over salads or cooked grains.

½ cup (125 ml) **pureed fresh tomatoes or canned tomatoes**

3 tablespoons (45 ml) **reduced-sodium tamari**

2 tablespoons (30 ml) **balsamic vinegar or apple cider vinegar**

2 tablespoons (30 ml) **peeled and grated fresh ginger**

2 cloves garlic, crushed

1 teaspoon (5 ml) **ground turmeric**

Put all the ingredients in a blender and process until smooth. Stored in a sealed container in the refrigerator, the marinade will keep for 3 weeks.

Leftover marinade can be refrigerated and used for other recipes. If you're a fan of ginger, feel free to double the amount. If you like heat, add a pinch of cayenne.

Per 2 tablespoons
(30 ml):
calories: 15
protein: 1 g
fat: 0 g
carbohydrate: 3 g
dietary fiber: 0 g
calcium: 7 mg
sodium: 301 mg

Walnut Pesto

MAKES 1 CUP
(250 ML)

This is an excellent sauce for bean pasta or rice, and it also makes a tasty dip for raw vegetables. Walnuts are rich in omega-3 fatty acids, which can go rancid over time, so make sure the walnuts you use are fresh. Store walnuts, as well as other nuts and seeds, in the refrigerator or freezer.

- **1 cup (250 ml) walnuts**
- **4 cups (1 L) fresh basil leaves, lightly packed**
- **2 tablespoons (30 ml) water**
- **2 tablespoons (30 ml) lemon juice**
- **2 tablespoons (30 ml) tamari**
- **2 cloves garlic, crushed**
- **⅛ teaspoon (0.5 ml) ground black pepper**

Put the walnuts in a food processor and pulse or process until finely chopped. Add the basil, water, lemon juice, tamari, garlic, and pepper and process until smooth, stopping occasionally to scrape down the work bowl. Serve immediately or store in a sealed container in the freezer.

VARIATION: Replace the walnuts with an equal amount of pine nuts.

Per 2 tablespoons (30 ml): calories: 106 protein: 3 g fat: 10 g carbohydrate: 4 g dietary fiber: 2 g calcium: 50 mg sodium: 252 mg

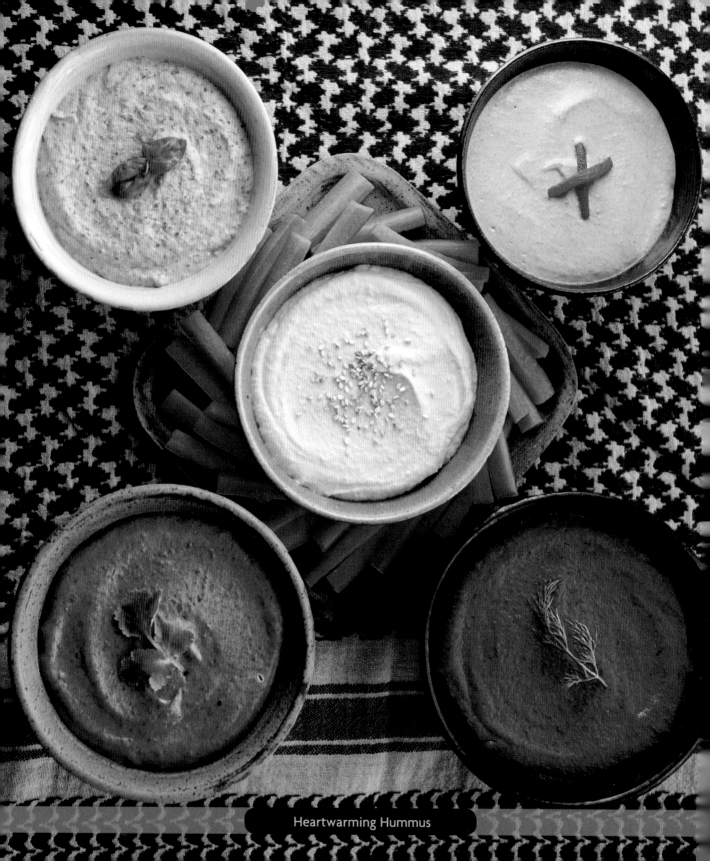

Heartwarming Hummus

Heartwarming Hummus

MAKES 2 CUPS (500 ML)

Hummus is magical. It can balance blood glucose levels and is an outstanding source of protein. In addition, it's quite versatile. Hummus can take the central position on a colorful platter of raw vegetables (see page 91), provide a quick snack day or night, or be turned into a salad dressing (see page 107). So keep it handy, near the front of the fridge.

1½ cups (375 ml) cooked or canned chickpeas, drained and rinsed

¼ cup (60 ml) tahini

¼ cup (60 ml) lemon juice

2 cloves garlic, crushed

½ teaspoon (2 ml) ground cumin

½ teaspoon (2 ml) salt

Pinch cayenne (optional)

⅓ cup (85 ml) water, as needed

Put the chickpeas, tahini, lemon juice, garlic, cumin, salt, and optional cayenne in a food processor and process until smooth, stopping occasionally to scrape down the work bowl. Add water as needed to achieve the desired consistency. Stored in a sealed container in the refrigerator, the hummus will keep for 5 days.

BLACK BEAN HUMMUS: Replace the chickpeas with an equal amount of black beans.

BLUSHING BEET HUMMUS: Omit the cumin. Add 1 boiled or roasted and chopped beet and 1 teaspoon (5 ml) dried dill weed.

CHEESY WHITE BEAN HUMMUS: Replace the chickpeas with an equal amount of cannellini, lima, or white beans. Add ¼ cup (60 ml) nutritional yeast flakes and ¼ cup (60 ml) jarred roasted red peppers.

GREEN GODDESS HUMMUS: Add ½–1 cup (125–250 ml) fresh herbs, such as basil, chives, cilantro, dill, or parsley, or a combination. Use additional herbs to garnish.

LIME HUMMUS: Replace the lemon juice with freshly squeezed lime juice.

Per ⅓ cup (85 ml):
calories: 136
protein: 5 g
fat: 6 g
carbohydrate: 17 g
dietary fiber: 4 g
calcium: 66 mg
sodium: 388 mg

RED-HOT HUMMUS: Add ½ teaspoon to 2 tablespoons (2–30 ml) chile paste or hot sauce, or ½–1 chipotle chile.

ROASTED RED PEPPER HUMMUS: Add ⅓ cup (85 ml) jarred roasted red peppers.

SUN-DRIED TOMATO HUMMUS: Put ½ cup (125 ml) sun-dried tomatoes in a heatproof bowl and cover with boiling water. Let soak for 30 minutes. Drain, reserving the soaking water. Add the tomatoes to the other ingredients before processing, and use the soaking water to thin the hummus as needed.

Red and Green Dip

MAKES 1.75 CUPS (425 ML)

Be sure to chop and stir in the fresh parsley by hand after processing the other ingredients; don't add it to the food processor. This will preserve the beautiful color of this dip.

1 cup (250 ml) **sun-dried tomatoes, soaked in warm water until soft and drained**

1 cup (250 ml) **Cashew Mayonnaise** (page 109)

½ cup (125 ml) **peeled and coarsely chopped cucumber**

1 teaspoon (5 ml) **light miso**

½ teaspoon (2 ml) **fresh or dried rosemary**

½ teaspoon (2 ml) **cayenne** (optional)

⅓ cup (85 ml) **minced fresh parsley or dill, lightly packed**

Put the tomatoes, mayonnaise, cucumber, miso, rosemary, and optional cayenne in a food processor and process until smooth, stopping occasionally to scrape down the work bowl. Transfer to a small bowl and stir in the parsley. Stored in a sealed container in the refrigerator, the dip will keep for 5 days.

Per ¼ cup (60 ml):
calories: 81
protein: 3 g
fat: 5 g
carbohydrate: 7 g
dietary fiber: 1 g
calcium: 18 mg
sodium: 182 mg

Tahini-Zucchini Dip

This bean-free dip has all the flavor of Middle Eastern hummus and is packed with bone-strengthening calcium. Enjoy it with crudités or spoon it into romaine lettuce boats and top with tomatoes and sprouts.

MAKES 1½ CUPS
(375 ML)

1 cup (250 ml) **peeled and chopped zucchini**

3½ tablespoons (52 ml) **lemon juice**

2 cloves **garlic, crushed**

1 teaspoon (5 ml) **paprika**

½ teaspoon (2 ml) **salt**

¼ teaspoon (1 ml) **ground cumin** (optional)

⅛ teaspoon (0.5 ml) **cayenne**

½ cup (125 ml) **tahini**

⅓ cup (85 ml) **sesame seeds, soaked in water for 4 hours, drained, and rinsed**

Put the zucchini, lemon juice, garlic, paprika, salt, optional cumin, and cayenne in a blender and process until smooth. Add the tahini and sesame seeds and process until smooth and creamy. Stored in a sealed container in the refrigerator, the dip will keep for 4 days.

This recipe can be made in a food processor if you don't have access to a blender, but the texture won't be as smooth and the sesame seeds will mostly remain whole.

Per ¼ cup (60 ml):
calories: 167
protein: 5 g
fat: 14 g
carbohydrate: 8 g
dietary fiber: 3 g
calcium: 169 mg
sodium: 225 mg

Brown Mushroom Gravy

MAKES 3¼ CUPS
(810 ML)

You might be surprised to discover that gravy made without fat can be incredibly delicious. This version is both fat-free and gluten-free. If you're not wild about mushrooms, omit them; the gravy will still be delicious.

2½ cups (625 ml) **water or vegetable broth**

2 cups (500 ml) **sliced mushrooms**

½ onion, **finely diced**

2 cloves garlic, crushed, **or 1 teaspoon (5 ml) garlic powder**

¼ cup (60 ml) **nutritional yeast flakes**

2 tablespoons (30 ml) **tamari**

1 tablespoon (15 ml) **light or dark miso**

2 teaspoons (10 ml) **poultry seasoning** (see Tip)

¼ teaspoon (1 ml) **ground black pepper**

2 tablespoons (30 ml) **cornstarch, or ¼ cup (60 ml) arrowroot starch**

¼ cup (60 ml) **cold water**

If you don't have poultry seasoning on hand, use ½ teaspoon (2 ml) each of dried parsley, sage, rosemary, and thyme.

Put ¼ cup (60 ml) of the water and the mushrooms, onion, and garlic in a medium saucepan. Cook over medium heat, stirring occasionally, until the vegetables are soft, about 10 minutes. Add more water if needed to prevent sticking.

Add the remaining 2¼ cups (550 ml) of the water and the nutritional yeast, tamari, miso, poultry seasoning, and pepper. Decrease the heat to low and cook, stirring occasionally, for 5 minutes.

Put the cornstarch in a small bowl. Add the cold water and stir to form a thick paste. Add ¼ cup (60 ml) of the hot liquid from the saucepan to the starch mixture and stir until smooth. Pour into the saucepan and bring to a boil over medium-high heat, whisking constantly. Cook, whisking constantly, until the gravy thickens, about 1 minute.

VARIATION: Replace ½ cup (125 ml) of the water with white wine.

Per ¼ cup (60 ml):

calories: 31

protein: 2 g

fat: 0 g

carbohydrate: 5 g

dietary fiber: 1 g

calcium: 13 mg

sodium: 310 mg

Savory Chickpea Gravy

U se all the seasonings listed in the recipe or just some of them. Either way, you will still have a lovely, aromatic, and protein-rich gravy.

MAKES 3 CUPS
(750 ML)

2 cups (500 ml) water, plus more as needed

1 onion, finely diced

1 cup (250 ml) cooked or canned chickpeas, drained and rinsed

¼ cup (60 ml) tamari

4 cloves garlic, crushed

2 tablespoons (30 ml) cornstarch or arrowroot starch

½ teaspoon (2 ml) dried parsley

½ teaspoon (2 ml) dried sage

½ teaspoon (2 ml) dried rosemary

½ teaspoon (2 ml) dried thyme

½ teaspoon (2 ml) ground celery seeds

½ teaspoon (2 ml) ground black pepper

Put 2 tablespoons (30 ml) of the water and the onion in a medium saucepan. Cook over medium heat, stirring occasionally, until the onion is soft, about 5 minutes. Add a little more water if needed to prevent sticking.

Put 1 cup (250 ml) of the water and the chickpeas, tamari, and garlic in a blender and process until smooth. Add the remaining water and the cornstarch, parsley, sage, rosemary, thyme, celery seeds, and pepper and process until well combined. Pour into the saucepan with the onion and bring to a boil over medium-high heat, whisking constantly. Cook, whisking constantly, until the gravy thickens, about 1 minute.

Per ¼ cup (60 ml):
calories: 38
protein: 2 g
fat: 0.3 g
carbohydrate: 7 g
dietary fiber: 1 g
calcium: 15 mg
sodium: 397 mg

Cheesy Cashew Red Pepper Sauce

MAKES 2 CUPS
(500 ML)

This sauce is fabulous on steamed vegetables, patties, or loaves and makes a fine filling for celery sticks. Stir it into soups or stews just before serving to impart a creamy texture and cheesy taste. Soaking the cashews prior to blending increases the availability of their minerals and helps to ensure a smooth sauce.

2 cups (500 ml) water

½ cup (125 ml) raw cashews, soaked for 2 hours, drained, and rinsed

1 fresh or roasted red bell pepper, seeded and coarsely chopped

3 tablespoons (45 ml) cornstarch or arrowroot starch

3 tablespoons (45 ml) nutritional yeast flakes

2 tablespoons (30 ml) lemon juice

2 cloves garlic, crushed, or ¾ teaspoon (4 ml) garlic powder and
    ¾ teaspoon (4 ml) onion powder

½ teaspoon (2 ml) salt

For an extra-silky sauce, process it again in the blender just before serving.

Put all the ingredients in a blender and process until smooth and creamy. Pour into a medium saucepan and bring almost to a boil over medium-high heat. Immediately decrease the heat to medium and cook, stirring or whisking frequently, until thickened, about 5 minutes. Stored in a sealed container in the refrigerator, the sauce will keep for 5 days.

CHEESY CASHEW RED PEPPER DIP OR DRESSING: Thin with additional lemon juice and/or water, 1 teaspoon (5 ml) at a time, until the desired consistency is achieved.

CHEESY SUNFLOWER RED PEPPER SAUCE: Replace the cashews with an equal amount of raw sunflower seeds.

Per ¼ cup (60 ml):
calories: 66
protein: 2 g
fat: 4 g
carbohydrate: 7 g
dietary fiber: 1 g
calcium: 6 mg
sodium: 150 mg

Cranberry Crunch Relish

MAKES 2¾ CUPS
(675 ML)

Cranberries are a rich source of antioxidants and vitamins, particularly vitamin C. This unique condiment makes a terrific topping for hot or cold breakfast cereals and also works as a sweet relish to accompany savory dishes, such as veggie loaves (see page 144) and burgers or stuffed squash (see page 140). Try layering it with Cashew-Pear Cream (page 171) for a delightful dessert parfait.

12 ounces (340 g) **fresh cranberries**

1 tablespoon (15 ml) **orange zest**

1 large navel orange, peeled (after zesting) **and coarsely chopped**

1 sweet apple, coarsely chopped

1 teaspoon (5 ml) **ground cinnamon**

Pinch ground cloves

Put all the ingredients in a food processor and pulse just until mixed but still chunky. Stored in a covered container in the refrigerator, the relish will keep for 4 days.

Per ¼ cup (60 ml):
calories: 36
protein: 0 g
fat: 0.1 g
carbohydrate: 8 g
dietary fiber: 2 g
calcium: 15 mg
sodium: 0 mg

8

VEGETABLES AND SIDE DISHES

Steamed Greens

MAKES 2 CUPS
(500 ML)

Aim to include dark leafy greens three times per day, either on their own or as part of another dish. You can even serve greens for breakfast or enjoy them as a side dish or snack.

4 cups (1 L) stemmed and chopped dark leafy greens (such as kale, collard greens, or mustard greens), **packed**

2 cloves garlic, crushed (optional)

1½ teaspoons (7 ml) balsamic vinegar, other vinegar, or balsamic reduction

1 teaspoon (5 ml) tamari

¼ teaspoon (1 ml) crushed red pepper flakes (optional)

2 teaspoons (10 ml) seeds (such as hemp, pumpkin, sesame, or sunflower seeds)

Serve the greens drizzled with Lemon-Tahini Dressing (page 104) or another favorite dressing in addition to or in place of the garlic, vinegar, tamari, and crushed red pepper flakes.

Steam the greens and garlic until the greens are wilted, 3–6 minutes (large, tough leaves will take longer than small, tender leaves). Alternatively, put the greens in a large bowl and pour boiling water over them; let them sit until softened, 1–2 minutes, then drain.

Transfer the greens to a medium bowl and add the vinegar, tamari, and optional red pepper flakes and toss or stir until well distributed. Garnish with the seeds. Serve warm, room temperature, or cold. Stored in a covered container in the refrigerator, the greens will keep for 2 days.

MAIN-DISH GREENS: To turn the greens into a main dish, add cubed tofu (plain, baked, or smoked), cubed or sliced tempeh, or cooked or canned beans, along with cubed cooked beets, butternut squash, or sweet potatoes.

VARIATIONS: Add peeled and grated fresh ginger or fresh or dried herbs, such as basil or dill.

Per 1 cup (250 ml):
calories: 98
protein: 6 g
fat: 1 g
carbohydrate: 16 g
dietary fiber: 3 g
calcium: 188 mg
sodium: 227 mg

Note: Analysis done with kale and pumpkin seeds.

KALE HOLLY WREATH

MAKES 6–8 SERVINGS This simple yet elegant dish is perfect for the holiday season and adds color and a festive touch any time of the year. Plus, it's an excellent source of vitamins A and C and a good source of calcium, iron, potassium, and vitamin B₆. If you prefer, use tiny cherry tomatoes or red currant tomatoes in place of the red bell pepper.

Double or triple the recipe for Steamed Greens (page 121), using kale. Instead of seeds, use 1 red bell pepper, finely diced. Arrange the seasoned kale on a large platter in the shape of a wreath by pushing the kale toward the edges of the platter, leaving a clean, open space in the center. Sprinkle the kale with the red bell pepper so the pieces look like holly berries.

Red Cabbage and Apples

MAKES 4 CUPS
(1 L)

This healthier version of a classic cabbage dish is rich in color and flavor but free of fat and sugar. Serve it alongside veggie loaves (see page 144) or patties or let it grace your table at holiday meals.

½ cup (125 ml) **water or vegetable broth**

1 onion, diced

4 cloves garlic, crushed

4 cups (1 L) thinly sliced red cabbage

2 red apples, chopped

¼ teaspoon (1 ml) ground allspice, cloves, or nutmeg, or whole or ground caraway seeds

½ teaspoon (2 ml) salt

¼ cup (60 ml) apple cider vinegar

Freshly ground black pepper

Per 1 cup (250 ml):
calories: 78
protein: 2 g
fat: 0.3 g
carbohydrate: 20 g
dietary fiber: 4 g
calcium: 50 mg
sodium: 320 mg

Put the water, onion, and garlic in a large saucepan over medium heat and cook, stirring occasionally, until the onion is soft, about 5 minutes. Add the cabbage, apples, allspice, and salt. Cover and cook, stirring occasionally, until the cabbage is tender, about 20 minutes. Add the vinegar and pepper to taste and cook uncovered, stirring occasionally, for 3 minutes. Serve hot, warm, or room temperature.

Mashed Rutabaga, Carrots, and Parsnips

MAKES 4 CUPS

(1 L)

Some people confuse rutabagas and turnips or use them interchangeably. Turnips are white and have more bite than rutabagas, which are yellowish, larger, and sweeter. If you prefer, you can replace the rutabaga with turnips in this recipe.

½ cup (125 ml) **fortified unsweetened soy milk or other
    nondairy milk**

½ cup (125 ml) **raw cashews**

2 cups (500 ml) **peeled and chopped rutabaga** (about ½ medium
    rutabaga)

3 **carrots, peeled if desired and chopped**

2 **parsnips, peeled if desired and chopped**

⅛ teaspoon (0.5 ml) **ground nutmeg**

¼ teaspoon (1 ml) **salt**

Freshly ground black pepper

Put the milk and cashews in a blender and process into a smooth cream. Set aside.

Put the rutabaga, carrots, and parsnips in a large saucepan. Cover with water and bring to a boil over medium-high heat. Decrease the heat to medium and cook until the vegetables break apart easily with a fork, 30–45 minutes. Drain and return the vegetables to the saucepan.

Add the cashew cream, nutmeg, and salt and mash with a fork or potato masher until the vegetables are as smooth or chunky as you like. Season with pepper to taste.

Per 1 cup (250 ml):
calories: 203
protein: 6 g
fat: 9 g
carbohydrate: 30 g
dietary fiber: 7 g
calcium: 124 mg
sodium: 212 mg

Asian Green Beans

MAKES 4 CUPS
(1 L)

Green beans are a popular vegetable, even when they're served plain. Try this recipe and give them a little pizazz.

Per 1 cup (250 ml):
calories: 60
protein: 3 g
fat: 2 g
carbohydrate: 9 g
dietary fiber: 4 g
calcium: 60 mg
sodium: 95 mg

1 pound (454 g) green beans, trimmed

1 tablespoon (15 ml) tahini

1 tablespoon (15 ml) rice vinegar

1 tablespoon (15 ml) peeled and grated fresh ginger

1 teaspoon (5 ml) tamari

1 clove garlic, crushed

Steam the green beans until tender-crisp, 5–7 minutes. While the green beans are cooking, put the tahini, vinegar, ginger, tamari, and garlic in a medium bowl and stir to combine. Add the green beans and toss to coat. Serve hot, warm, or room temperature.

Steamed Vegetables with Cheesy Cashew Red Pepper Sauce

MAKES 4 SERVINGS

A delicious sauce makes any vegetable more appealing. In addition to the recommendations below, also try the sauce on baked potatoes, sweet potatoes, or your favorite veggies.

Per serving:
calories: 190
protein: 10 g
fat: 8 g
carbohydrate: 23 g
dietary fiber: 7 g
calcium: 66 mg
sodium: 304 mg

Note: Analysis done with asparagus.

2 pounds (900 g) asparagus, broccoli, broccolini, cauliflower, green beans, and/or Romanesco broccoli

2 cups (500 ml) Cheesy Cashew Red Pepper Sauce (page 118), hot

Cut the vegetables into uniform pieces and steam until tender-crisp. Transfer to a serving bowl and top with the hot sauce.

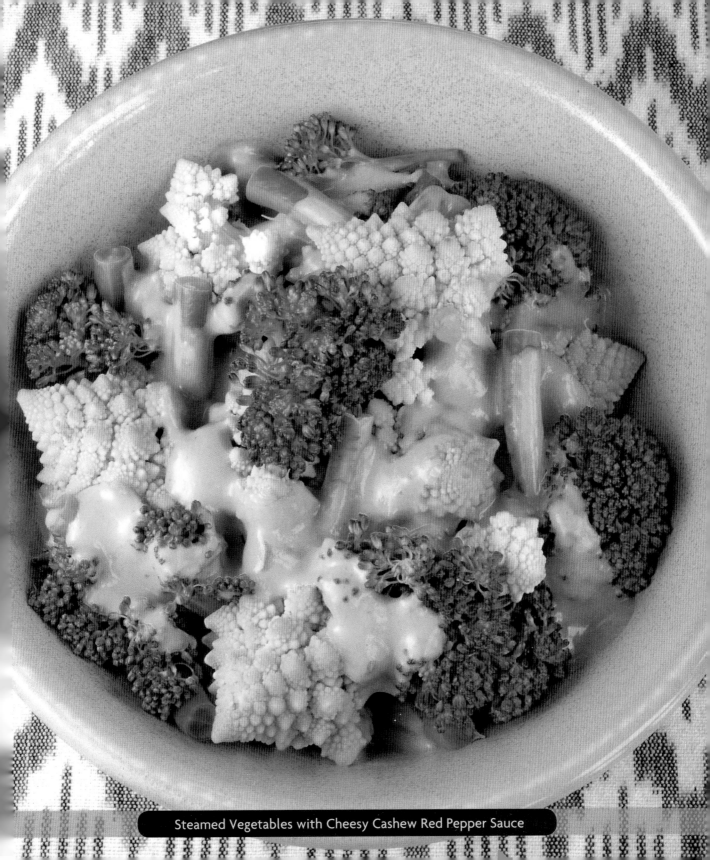

Steamed Vegetables with Cheesy Cashew Red Pepper Sauce

Ratatouille

MAKES 4½ CUPS
(1.125 L),
4 SERVINGS

What a fun dish to make! Layer these summer vegetables in a big skillet before you turn on the heat. Your reward will be a flavorful medley that's ready to serve right out of the pan.

⅓ cup (85 ml) **water**

1⅔ cups (415 ml) **thinly sliced onions** (cut into crescents)

⅓ cup (75 ml) **minced garlic**

1⅔ cups (415 ml) **red, orange, or yellow bell pepper strips**

2 cups (500 ml) **sliced mushrooms**

3 cups (750 ml) **sliced zucchini**

3 cups (750 ml) **peeled and cubed eggplant**

4 **Roma tomatoes, sliced**

1 teaspoon (5 ml) **dried basil**

1 teaspoon (5 ml) **dried oregano**

1 teaspoon (5 ml) **dried rosemary**

1 teaspoon (5 ml) **dried thyme**

½ teaspoon (2 ml) **salt**

½ teaspoon (2 ml) **ground black pepper**

Put the water in a large skillet. Layer each of the vegetables in the pan in the order listed, sprinkling some of the herbs, salt, and pepper over each layer. Cover and cook over medium heat for 15 minutes. Stir and cook uncovered for 10 minutes longer. Serve hot or room temperature.

MAIN-DISH RATATOUILLE: Add 1½ cups (375 ml) cooked or canned chickpeas during the final 10 minutes of cooking.

RATATOUILLE WITH SPINACH: Add 4 cups (1 L) spinach, lightly packed, during the final 10 minutes of cooking.

Per serving:
calories: 108
protein: 5 g
fat: 0.8 g
carbohydrate: 24 g
dietary fiber: 7 g
calcium: 93 mg
sodium: 318 mg

Baked Squash Casserole

MAKES 4 CUPS (1 L)

Despite its relatively high carbohydrate content, winter squash has a fairly low glycemic index of about 51. This means its carbohydrate is released more slowly into the bloodstream than most other starchy vegetables. As a bonus, it's loaded with a variety of carotenoids and antioxidants.

4 cups (1 L) **peeled and cubed winter squash** (see Tip)

6 tablespoons (100 ml) **orange juice with pulp** (juice from about 2 oranges)

2 cups (500 ml) **bite-sized fresh or frozen pineapple chunks**

¼ teaspoon (1 ml) **salt** (optional)

Preheat the oven to 350 F. Put in the ingredients in a medium casserole dish and stir until well combined. Cover and bake for 30 minutes. Stir well, cover, and bake for 30 minutes longer, or until the squash is soft.

Use acorn, butternut, hubbard, or any other orange-fleshed winter squash.

Per 1 cup (250 ml):
calories: 105
protein: 2 g
fat: 0.4 g
carbohydrate: 26 g
dietary fiber: 3 g
calcium: 50 mg
sodium: 9 mg

Brussels Sprouts with Lemon and Dill

MAKES 3 CUPS
(750 ML)

Brussels sprouts are one of the superstars of the cruciferous family, whose members are well recognized for their cancer-fighting properties. Brussels sprouts are loaded with vitamins and minerals and are an exceptional source of vitamins C and K.

4 cups (1 L) **halved Brussels sprouts**

¼ cup (60 ml) **water**

3 tablespoons (45 ml) **slivered almonds**

Juice of 1 lemon

¼ cup (60 ml) **minced fresh dill, or 1 tablespoon** (15 ml) **dried dill weed**

1 teaspoon (5 ml) **light miso**

Put the Brussels sprouts and water in a medium saucepan. Cover and cook over medium-high heat for 10 minutes. Decrease the heat to medium-low. Add the almonds, lemon juice, and dill and cook uncovered for 2 minutes. Remove from the heat and stir in the miso, mixing it well with the liquid in the bottom of the pan. Stir to evenly coat the Brussels sprouts. Let sit for 5–10 minutes before serving to allow the flavors to blend. Serve hot, room temperature, or cold.

Per 1 cup (250 ml):
calories: 95
protein: 6 g
fat: 4 g
carbohydrate: 13 g
dietary fiber: 5 g
calcium: 68 mg
sodium: 112 mg

Spicy Bok Choy

Loaded with antioxidants, bok choy is also rich in calcium, folate, potassium, and vitamins A, C, and K.

MAKES 3½ CUPS (875 ML)

1 tablespoon (15 ml) peeled and grated fresh ginger

1 teaspoon (5 ml) ground coriander

1 teaspoon (5 ml) crushed yellow mustard seeds

1 teaspoon (5 ml) ground turmeric

½ teaspoon (2 ml) chili powder or hot sauce (see Tip)

1 head bok choy, chopped, or 6 cups (1.5 L) chopped green cabbage

1 large onion, chopped

¼ cup (60 ml) water

3 cloves garlic, crushed

¼ cup (60 ml) chopped walnuts

2 tablespoons (30 ml) apple cider vinegar

¼ teaspoon (1 ml) salt (optional)

Ground black pepper

Add more or less chili powder to suit your taste.

Put the ginger, coriander, mustard seeds, turmeric, and chili powder in a medium saucepan and stir to combine. Cook over medium heat, stirring constantly, for 1 minute.

Add the bok choy, onion, water, and garlic. Cover and cook, stirring occasionally, until the vegetables are tender, 10–15 minutes. Add the walnuts and vinegar and stir to combine. Add the optional salt and season with pepper to taste. Cover and cook until heated through, about 1 minute.

Per 1¾ cups (435 ml):
calories: 198
protein: 8 g
fat: 11 g
carbohydrate: 23 g
dietary fiber: 5 g
calcium: 290 mg
sodium: 169 mg

9

MAIN DISHES

The Big Easy Bowl

MAKES 1 SERVING

This simple dish will sustain your energy wonderfully between meals. If you prefer, replace any of the vegetables with your favorites or with any leftover veggies that you have on hand.

¾ cup (185 ml) cooked hulled or pot barley, brown rice, Kamut berries, quinoa, spelt berries, or other whole grain

1 cup (250 ml) chopped spinach, lightly packed

1 cup (250 ml) cooked or canned beans (any kind), drained and rinsed, or 4 slices Marinated Tofu (page 135) or smoked tofu

½ cup (125 ml) grated raw beet or chopped cooked beet

½ cup (125 ml) grated carrot

2 tablespoons (30 ml) raw or roasted pumpkin seeds or almonds

3 tablespoons (45 ml) salad dressing of choice (see pages 104–109)

Put the grain in a bowl. Add the spinach, beans, beet, and carrot. Sprinkle the seeds over the top and drizzle with the dressing.

VARIATION: Add 2 cups (500 ml) hot steamed vegetables, such as thinly sliced carrots or bell peppers, broccoli or cauliflower florets, pea pods, sliced asparagus, and/or stemmed and chopped kale.

For a packed lunch, layer all the ingredients in a mason jar and seal with a lid. To reduce calories, decrease the amount of cooked grain to ½ cup (125 ml).

Per serving:
calories: 564
protein: 28 g
fat: 13 g
carbohydrate: 88 g
dietary fiber: 27 g
calcium: 116 mg
sodium: 104 mg

Note: Analysis done with black beans, hulled barley, and raw pumpkin seeds. It doesn't include salad dressing.

African Chickpea Stew

MAKES 6 CUPS
(1.5 L)

The creamy sauce in this nutrition-packed stew comes from peanut butter. If you prefer, use almond butter instead.

4 cups (1 L) water or vegetable broth

2 cups (500 ml) peeled and diced sweet potatoes

1½ cups (375 ml) cooked or canned chickpeas, drained and rinsed

1 onion, chopped

½ cup (125 ml) brown rice

2 cloves garlic, crushed

½ teaspoon (2 ml) salt

¼ cup (60 ml) peanut butter or almond butter

2 cups (500 ml) stemmed and chopped collard greens or kale, packed

2 tablespoons (30 ml) lemon juice

Tamari (optional)

Chili sauce or hot sauce (optional)

Put the water, sweet potatoes, chickpeas, onion, rice, garlic, and salt in a large saucepan and bring to a boil over medium-high heat. Decrease the heat to medium-low and cook, stirring occasionally, for 45 minutes.

Put the peanut butter in a small bowl. Add ½ cup of the liquid from the stew and stir well to make a smooth paste. Stir into the stew along with the collard greens and cook for 5 minutes. Add the lemon juice and stir until well combined. Season with optional tamari and chili sauce.

Per 1 cup (250 ml):
calories: 262
protein: 9 g
fat: 7 g
carbohydrate: 43 g
dietary fiber: 6 g
calcium: 81 mg
sodium: 220 mg

Sweet Potato and Black Bean Chili

MAKES 4½ CUPS
(1 L)

This chili has great visual appeal. To complement the contrasting colors and textures, serve it with a big green salad. Double the recipe if desired.

½ cup (125 ml) **water or vegetable broth**

1½ cups (375 ml) **cooked or canned black beans, rinsed and drained**

1 cup (250 ml) **orange sweet potato, peeled and diced**

1 cup (250 ml) **canned diced tomatoes**

1 cup (250 ml) **fresh, frozen, or canned corn**

½ **onion, chopped**

½ **green, orange, or red bell pepper, diced**

1½ teaspoons (7 ml) **chili powder or hot sauce**

2 cloves **garlic, crushed**

½ teaspoon (2 ml) **salt**

¼ teaspoon (1 ml) **ground black pepper** (optional)

¼ teaspoon (1 ml) **smoked paprika** (optional)

Pinch cayenne (optional)

1 **avocado, cubed**

2 tablespoons (30 ml) **lime juice, or lime wedges, as desired**

Put the water, beans, sweet potatoes, tomatoes, corn, onion, bell pepper, chili powder, garlic, salt, optional pepper, optional paprika, and optional cayenne in a medium saucepan and bring to a boil over medium-high heat. Decrease the heat to medium-low and cook, stirring occasionally, until the sweet potato is soft, about 20 minutes. Serve with the avocado and lime juice on the side.

Per 1½ cups (375 ml):
calories: 320
protein: 11 g
fat: 11 g
carbohydrate: 49 g
dietary fiber: 15 g
calcium: 80 mg
sodium: 440 mg

Vegetable Kabobs

MAKES 6 LARGE
KABOBS

These kabobs can be cooked on a grill or baked in the oven. If you grill, use a low temperature and avoid blackening the food. The marinade is absorbed by the tofu, providing a burst of flavor. Serve it with cooked brown rice or another whole grain on the side.

18 cubes extra-firm tofu (each cube about 1 inch/3 cm), **marinated for at least 6 hours** (see Tofu or Tempeh Marinade, page 110)

12 mushrooms, quartered

12 squares red bell pepper (each square about 1 inch/3 cm)

12 thick slices zucchini

12 cherry tomatoes

12 pieces red onion (each piece about 1 inch/3 cm)

Thread the tofu and vegetables tightly on six 10- or 12-inch (25–28 cm) metal or soaked bamboo skewers, alternating each item. Drizzle any extra marinade over the skewers. Cook on an indoor or outdoor grill or put on a baking sheet six inches (15 cm) below the broiler for 10 minutes, turning once. Avoid blackening the food.

VARIATION: Include 12 pineapple chunks and/or other vegetables.

Per kabob:
calories: 123
protein: 13 g
fat: 5 g
carbohydrate: 9 g
dietary fiber: 3 g
calcium: 126 mg
sodium: 382 mg

Marinated Tofu

MAKES 8 SLICES,

4 SERVINGS

Tofu is porous and readily absorbs the flavors of seasonings and marinades, making it very versatile. Look for tofu that's high in calcium. Slices can be served atop salads or alongside vegetables to make a low-calorie, high-protein meal.

1 block (16 ounces/450 g) **firm or extra-firm tofu**

⅞ cup (220 ml) **Tofu or Tempeh Marinade** (page 110)

Cut the tofu into thin (¼-inch/1-cm) slices. Arrange the slices in a single layer in one or two glass baking dishes. Evenly pour the marinade over the tofu. Cover and let marinate in the refrigerator for at least 6 hours.

To cook on the stove top, remove the tofu from the marinade (see Tip). For stovetop cooking, use a large nonstick skillet or a regular skillet misted with cooking spray. Cook in batches over medium heat until lightly brown on both sides, turning once. To microwave, use a microwave-safe plate and cook on high until the tofu just begins to brown. To bake, preheat the oven to 350 degrees F (175 degrees C). Line a baking sheet with parchment paper or a silicone baking mat or mist it with cooking spray. Arrange the slices on the prepared baking sheet in a single layer and bake until they just begin to brown, about 15 minutes.

MARINATED TEMPEH: Replace the tofu with 2 packages (8 ounces/240 g per package) tempeh, sliced or cubed.

About one-quarter of the marinade will be left over and can be used for other recipes. Stored in a covered container in the refrigerator, the leftover marinade will keep for 3 weeks.

Per serving (2 slices):
calories: 130
protein: 15 g
fat: 7 g
carbohydrate: 5 g
dietary fiber: 2 g
calcium: 144 mg
sodium: 410 mg

Note: Analysis done with reduced-sodium tamari.

The Three Sisters Go Green

MAKES 6 CUPS
(1.5 L)

The three sisters—squash, beans, and corn—were the main crops of several Native American nations. These plants benefit each other, so they were grown close together. Not surprisingly, this companionable trio benefits people as well.

Vary the seasonings to suit your taste. You can replace butternut with other small winter squashes, but those may be more difficult to peel.

1 cup (250 ml) **water or vegetable broth**

3 cups (750 ml) **peeled and cubed butternut squash**

1 onion, diced

2 cloves garlic, crushed

1½ cups (375 ml) **fresh or canned diced tomatoes**

1½ cups (375 ml) **cooked or canned pinto beans or pink beans, drained and rinsed**

1 cup (250 ml) **frozen or canned corn**

1 green chile, minced (optional)

1 teaspoon (5 ml) **ground cumin**

1 teaspoon (5 ml) **dried oregano**

½ teaspoon (2 ml) **salt** (optional)

¼ teaspoon (1 ml) **ground black pepper**

2 cups (500 ml) **stemmed and thinly sliced kale or other dark leafy greens, packed**

2 tablespoons (30 ml) **minced fresh cilantro or parsley**

Put the water, squash, onion, and garlic in a large saucepan and bring to a boil over medium-high heat. Decrease the heat to medium and cook, stirring occasionally, until the squash is tender, about 20 minutes. Add the tomatoes, beans, corn, optional chile, cumin, oregano, optional salt, and pepper and cook, stirring occasionally, for 15 minutes. Add the kale and cook, stirring occasionally, until the kale is tender, 3–5 minutes. Sprinkle the cilantro over the top just before serving.

Per 1 cup (250 ml):
calories: 156
protein: 7 g
fat: 1 g
carbohydrate: 34 g
dietary fiber: 9 g
calcium: 131 mg
sodium: 235 mg

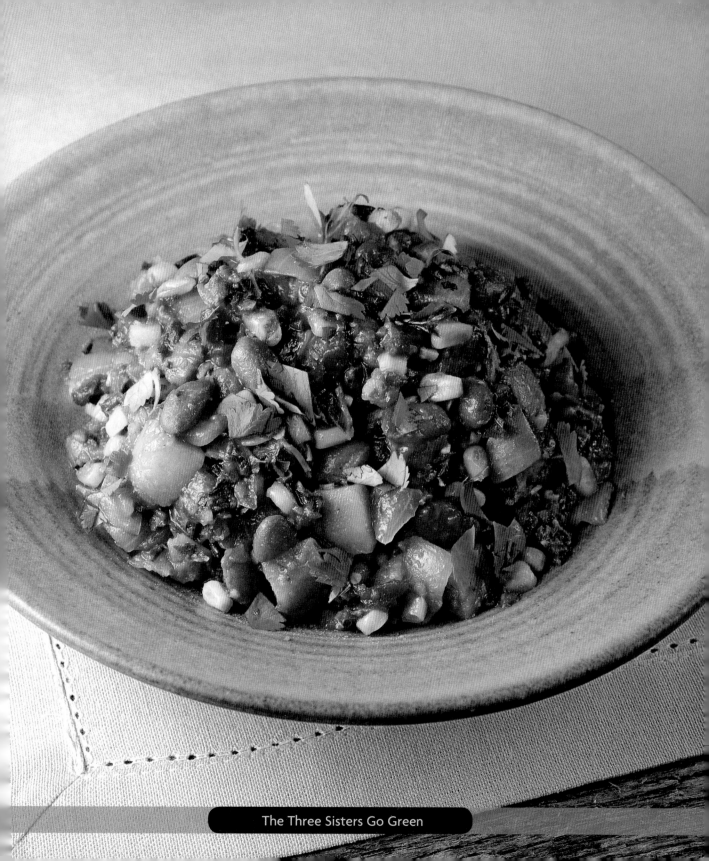

The Three Sisters Go Green

Veggie Tomato Pasta

MAKES 6½ CUPS
(1.63 L)

This vegetable-rich sauce is packed with protective phytochemicals. Serve it over any type of pasta, preferably one that's made with legumes. For added flavor and nutrition, top it with Cheesy Cashew Red Pepper Sauce (page 118), veggie meatballs, or a sprinkle of nutritional yeast.

Protein-rich bean pastas will help maintain your blood glucose level between meals. Look for ones made with adzuki beans, black beans, chickpeas, red lentils, or other legumes.

1 can (28 ounces/830 ml) **stewed tomatoes, or 3½ cups (830 ml) chopped fresh tomatoes**

1 cup (250 ml) **water**

1 can (6 ounces/128 ml) **tomato paste**

1 **onion, diced**

1 stalk **broccoli, chopped**

1 small **zucchini, sliced or grated**

1 **carrot, sliced diagonally**

1 cup (250 ml) **sliced mushrooms**

3 cloves **garlic, crushed**

½ cup (125 ml) **red, orange, yellow, or green bell pepper, diced**

4 teaspoons (20 ml) **Italian seasoning, or 2 teaspoons (10 ml) dried basil and 2 teaspoons (10 ml) dried oregano**

½ teaspoon (2 ml) **salt** (optional)

Freshly ground black pepper

Crushed red pepper flakes or hot sauce (optional)

Cooked pasta (1 cup/250 ml per serving), **hot**

Per 1⅓ cups (415 ml):
calories: 408
protein: 25 g
fat: 3 g
carbohydrate: 76 g
dietary fiber: 18 g
calcium: 242 mg
sodium: 128 mg

Note: Analysis done with red lentil rotini.

Put the tomatoes, water, tomato paste, onion, broccoli, zucchini, carrot, mushrooms, garlic, bell pepper, and Italian seasoning in a large saucepan and stir to combine. Bring to a boil over medium-high heat, cover, decrease the heat to medium-low, and cook, stirring occasionally, for 45 minutes. Alternatively, put the ingredients in a slow cooker and cook on low for 6 hours or on high for 4 hours. Add the optional salt and season with pepper and optional red pepper flakes to taste. Serve hot over pasta.

VARIATIONS: Try other vegetables, such as chopped cauliflower, diced celery, stemmed and chopped kale, or chopped spinach, or use a combination of vegetables. For added protein (if you're not using a legume-based pasta), add 1–2 cups (250–500 ml) cooked lentils to the sauce.

Full-Meal Baked Potatoes or Sweet Potatoes

Dinner can be a cinch when you have potatoes or sweet potatoes on hand, especially if they've been cooked in advance. Whenever you bake something (such as Baked Apple-Spice Oatmeal, page 63, or Chewy Walnut Cookies, page 164), put some scrubbed potatoes in the oven at the same time. Alternatively, microwave them in the oven shortly before dinner, although they won't have the same flavor and texture as potatoes that have been oven-baked. There are many healthy options for toppings; we've listed a few to get your creative juices pumping.

OVEN METHOD: Preheat the oven to 375 degrees F (190 degrees C). Scrub the potatoes and pierce each of them three or four times with a knife or fork. Bake directly on the middle oven rack for 45 minutes, or until soft when gently squeezed (use an oven mitt!) or when a fork or skewer slides in easily.

MICROWAVE METHOD: Scrub the potatoes and pierce each of them three or four times with a knife or fork. Microwave on high for about 5 minutes, depending on the size of potatoes, until soft.

TO COMPLETE THE MEAL: Cut an X on top of each potato or sweet potato and top with any of the following:

- **Black beans, salsa, and several slices of avocado**
- **Sweet Potato and Black Bean Chili** (page 133)
- **Lemon-Tahini Dressing** (page 104) **or another dressing** (see pages 105–109); **serve with a soup or salad**
- **Steamed broccoli, cooked or canned beans, and Cheesy Cashew Red Pepper Sauce** (page 118)
- **Steamed vegetables, cooked or canned chickpeas, and Lemon-Tahini Dressing** (page 104)

Stuffed Winter Squash

MAKES 6 HEARTY
WEDGES OR 12
SMALLER WEDGES;
6 CUPS (1.5 L)
STUFFING

For some families or groups of friends, getting together to cook is one of the best parts of a celebration. Assembling this stuffing and baked squash can be a central activity for a day spent with the people you love. Serve the squash with Brown Mushroom Gravy (page 116) or Savory Chickpea Gravy (page 117), plus a big salad or a Kale Holly Wreath (page 122). It makes a lovely centerpiece.

1 large winter squash (about 5 pounds/2.267 kg; see Tip)

1½ cups (375 ml) cooked brown rice or quinoa

1½ cups (375 ml) cooked or canned lentils, drained and rinsed

½ onion, diced

2 stalks celery, diced

¼ cup (60 ml) water

2 cloves garlic, crushed

1 cup (250 ml) fresh, frozen, or canned corn

½ cup (125 ml) diced orange, red, or yellow bell pepper

½ cup (125 ml) sunflower seeds, pumpkin seeds, or chopped almonds or cashews

¼ cup (60 ml) chopped fresh parsley, lightly packed

1 teaspoon (5 ml) dried oregano

1 teaspoon (5 ml) dried thyme

½ teaspoon (2 ml) dried sage

2 tablespoons (30 ml) reduced-sodium tamari

⅛ teaspoon (0.5 ml) pepper

Per hearty wedge:
calories: 376
protein: 13 g
fat: 6 g
carbohydrate: 75 g
dietary fiber: 20 g
calcium: 197 mg
sodium: 461 mg

Note: Analysis done
with Hubbard squash.

Preheat the oven to 350 degrees F (175 degrees C). Pierce the top of the squash with a sharp knife held at a 45-degree angle. Push the knife blade away from your body, rotate the blade around top of squash, and remove the cone-shaped top piece. Remove any fibrous material from the cone and set the top aside. Remove the seeds and pulp from the cavity of the squash with a soup spoon. Put the squash and its top in a large baking pan and bake for 45 minutes. Remove from the oven and let cool in the pan for 15 minutes. Don't turn off the oven.

To make the stuffing, put the rice and lentils in a large bowl and set aside. Put the onion, celery, water, and garlic in a large saucepan and cook over medium heat, stirring frequently, for 5 minutes. Add to the rice and lentils along with the corn, bell pepper, sunflower seeds, parsley, oregano, thyme, sage, tamari, and pepper. Stir until well combined.

Spoon the stuffing into the cavity of the squash until it is full. Put the top on and bake for 45–60 minutes, or until a toothpick slides easily into the squash. Transfer to a serving platter and slice into wedges to serve.

STUFFED PEPPERS: Preheat the oven to 350 degrees F (175 degrees C). Cut a thin slice from the stem end of each pepper. Remove the seeds and membranes. If necessary, cut a thin slice off the bottoms to allow the peppers to stand upright. Arrange the peppers upright in a baking pan. Fill the peppers with the stuffing and decorate the tops with a slice of tomato and a little chopped fresh parsley. Bake for 45 minutes, or until the peppers are tender.

Choose a Hubbard or kabocha squash or a wide, squat butternut squash. Several smaller acorn squashes could work too. If the squash has thick flesh and a small cavity, the cooking time will be longer. If you have more stuffing than can fit in the squash, put it in a baking pan or loaf pan, sprinkle it with 2 tablespoons (30 ml) of water, cover, and put in the oven to heat through during the last 20 minutes of baking.

Tamale Pie

MAKES 8 SERVINGS

This is a tasty dish of Mexican-Spanish origin. Although any cornmeal will work for this recipe, we use coarsely ground whole-grain cornmeal because it's unrefined and retains the hull and germ. This means more nutrients and a lower glycemic index!

FILLING

1 onion, chopped

1 green bell pepper, diced

2 tablespoons (30 ml) **water or vegetable broth**

2 cloves garlic, crushed

1¾ cups (435 ml) **cooked or canned pinto beans, drained and rinsed**

1¾ cups (435 ml) **canned diced tomatoes**

1½ cups (375 ml) **frozen or canned corn**

1 cup (250 ml) **tomato sauce**

½ cup (125 ml) **sliced black olives**

⅓ cup (85 ml) **coarsely ground whole-grain cornmeal**

1 tablespoon (15 ml) **chili powder**

½ teaspoon (2 ml) **paprika**

Hot sauce (optional)

TOPPING

3 cups (750 ml) **water**

1 cup (250 ml) **coarsely ground whole-grain cornmeal**

¼ cup (60 ml) **nutritional yeast flakes**

¾ teaspoon (4 ml) **salt**

½ teaspoon (2 ml) **garlic powder**

Per serving:

calories: 208

protein: 10 g

fat: 3 g

carbohydrate: 40 g

dietary fiber: 9 g

calcium: 46 mg

sodium: 480 mg

To make the filling, put the onion, bell pepper, water, and garlic in a large saucepan. Cover and cook over medium heat until the onion is tender, about 5 minutes. Add the beans, tomatoes, corn, tomato sauce, olives, cornmeal, chili powder, and paprika and stir to combine. Increase the heat to medium-high and bring to a boil. Decrease the heat to medium-low, cover, and cook, stirring occasionally, for 15 minutes. Season with hot sauce if desired. While the bean mixture is cooking, prepare the topping.

To make the topping, put the water in a medium saucepan and bring to a boil over medium-high heat. Remove from the heat and stir in the cornmeal. Add the nutritional yeast, salt, and garlic powder and stir until well combined. Cook over medium-low heat, stirring almost constantly, until thick, about 15 minutes.

Preheat the oven to 375 degrees F (190 degrees C).

Transfer the bean mixture to a 13 x 9-inch (33 x 23-cm) casserole dish. Spread the topping evenly over the top. Bake for 30–40 minutes, until golden brown and bubbly. Serve hot.

VARIATION: For a cheesy flavor, fold ½ cup (125 ml) Cheesy Cashew Red Pepper Sauce (page 118) into the topping before spreading it over the bean mixture.

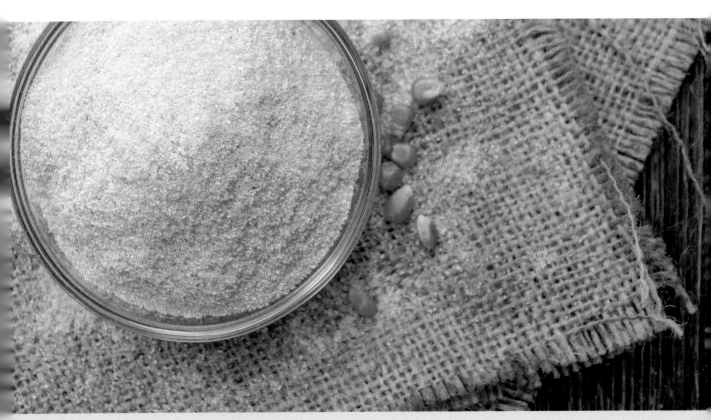

Lentil-Quinoa Nut Loaves

MAKES 2 LOAVES,
8 SERVINGS PER LOAF

A nut loaf is satisfying comfort food. Its high protein and fiber content contributes to satiety and helps stabilize blood sugar. Serve this homestyle version with a gravy (see pages 116 and 117), a side of Mashed Rutabaga, Carrots, and Parsnips (page 123), and green vegetables for a well-rounded meal.

½ cup (125 ml) **quinoa**

5⅔ cups (1.36 L) **water**

⅔ cup (165 ml) **pot barley** (see Tip)

⅔ cup (165 ml) **dried lentils** (see Tip)

1½ **large onions, finely chopped**

1 cup (250 ml) **walnuts, finely chopped**

3 **stalks celery, diced**

⅓ cup (85 ml) **ground flaxseeds**

¼ cup (60 ml) **chopped fresh parsley, lightly packed**

2 tablespoons (30 ml) **poultry seasoning** (see Tip, page 116)

⅔ cup (165 ml) **water**

1 cup (250 ml) **raw cashews**

⅓ cup (85 ml) **tamari**

6 **cloves garlic, chopped**

Freshly ground black pepper

Put the quinoa in a small saucepan. Add 1 cup (250 ml) of the water and bring to a boil over medium-high heat. Decrease the heat to low, cover, and cook until all the water is absorbed, 15–20 minutes. Remove from the heat and let cool.

Put the barley and lentils in a medium saucepan. Add 4 cups (1 L) of the water and bring to a boil over medium-high heat. Decrease the heat to low, cover, and cook until the lentils are soft, about 45 minutes. Drain.

Put the quinoa, barley mixture, onions, walnuts, celery, flaxseeds, parsley, and poultry seasoning in a large bowl and stir until well combined.

(continued on page 146)

Per serving:
calories: 191
protein: 8 g
fat: 10 g
carbohydrate: 21 g
dietary fiber: 7 g
calcium: 43 mg
sodium: 317 mg

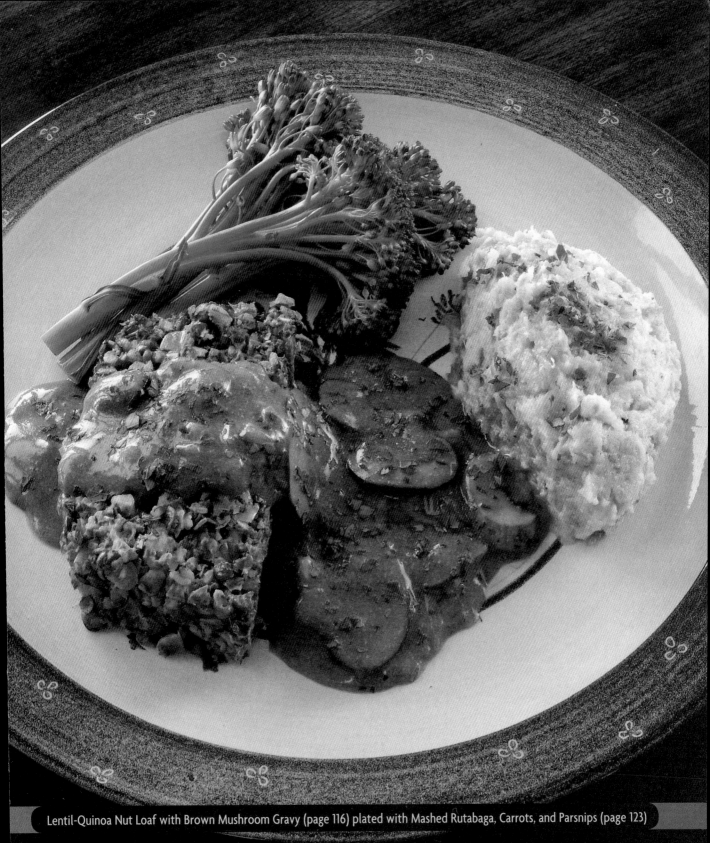

Lentil-Quinoa Nut Loaf with Brown Mushroom Gravy (page 116) plated with Mashed Rutabaga, Carrots, and Parsnips (page 123)

Put the remaining ⅔ cup (165 ml) of water and the cashews, tamari, and garlic in a blender and process until smooth. Pour into the quinoa mixture and stir until well combined. Season with pepper to taste.

Preheat the oven to 350 degrees F (175 degrees C). Lightly mist two loaf pans with cooking spray. Press the mixture evenly into the prepared loaf pans. Bake for 1–1½ hours, or until the loaves are slightly firm to the touch.

Pot barley is less processed than other kinds, so it's what we recommend, although any type of barley can be used in this recipe. Smaller lentils, such as French or beluga lentils, would be great, but regular brown or green lentils will work well too.

Moroccan Chickpeas

erve these savory chickpeas over your favorite whole grain, accompanied by a salad on the side.

MAKES 6 CUPS
(1.5 L)

4 cups (1 L) **peeled and cubed eggplant**

1 medium onion, **diced**

¼ cup (60 ml) **water, plus more as needed**

3 cloves garlic, **crushed**

3½ cups (875 ml) **crushed fresh or canned tomatoes**

2 cups (500 ml) **cooked or chickpeas, drained and rinsed**

¼ cup (60 ml) **raisins**

2 tablespoons (30 ml) **orange zest** (optional)

1 tablespoon (15 ml) **peeled and grated fresh ginger**

2 teaspoons (10 ml) **dried oregano**

½ teaspoon (2 ml) **salt**

½ teaspoon (2 ml) **ground cinnamon**

¼ teaspoon (1 ml) **ground black pepper**

Pinch **cayenne**

1 **bay leaf**

¼ cup (60 ml) **chopped fresh parsley, lightly packed**

Put the eggplant, onion, water, and garlic in a medium saucepan. Cook over medium heat, stirring occasionally, until the eggplant is soft, about 10 minutes. Add more water as needed to prevent sticking.

Add the tomatoes, chickpeas, raisins, optional orange zest, ginger, oregano, salt, cinnamon, pepper, cayenne, and bay leaf and bring to a boil over medium-high heat. Decrease the heat to medium and cook, stirring occasionally, for 10 minutes. Remove the bay leaf and stir in the parsley.

MEDITERRANEAN CHICKPEAS: Omit the raisins, orange zest, ginger, oregano, cinnamon, and cayenne. Stir in 1 tablespoon (15 ml) of Italian seasoning when adding the tomatoes.

Per 1 cup (250 ml):
calories: 189
protein: 9 g
fat: 2 g
carbohydrate: 39 g
dietary fiber: 11 g
calcium: 110 mg
sodium: 389 mg

Southwestern Stuffed Sweet Potatoes

MAKES 4 SERVINGS

Sweet potatoes are among the most nutritious and delicious of all the starchy vegetables. Use sweet potatoes with bright-orange flesh for this recipe. For a complete meal, serve the sweet potatoes with a green salad on the side.

4 sweet potatoes, scrubbed

1 onion, diced

1 small green bell pepper, diced

¼ cup (60 ml) water or vegetable broth

3 cloves garlic, crushed

1½ cups (375 ml) cooked or canned black beans, drained and rinsed

1½ cups (375 ml) fresh, frozen, or canned corn

1½ cups (375 ml) diced fresh tomatoes

1 teaspoon (5 ml) ground cumin

1 teaspoon (5 ml) chili powder

¼ teaspoon (1 ml) smoked paprika

¼ cup (60 ml) chopped fresh cilantro or parsley, lightly packed

2 tablespoons lime juice

¼ teaspoon (1 ml) salt (optional)

Freshly ground black pepper

Hot sauce (optional)

1 avocado, sliced

Cashew Mayonnaise (page 109; optional)

Preheat the oven to 350 degrees F (175 degrees C). Line a baking sheet or shallow baking pan with parchment paper or a silicone baking mat or mist it with cooking spray.

Pierce the sweet potatoes several times with a fork. Put them on the prepared baking sheet and bake for 45 minutes, or until soft.

(continued on page 150)

Per serving:

calories: 357

protein: 12 g

fat: 9 g

carbohydrate: 62 g

dietary fiber: 17 g

calcium: 98 mg

sodium: 341 mg

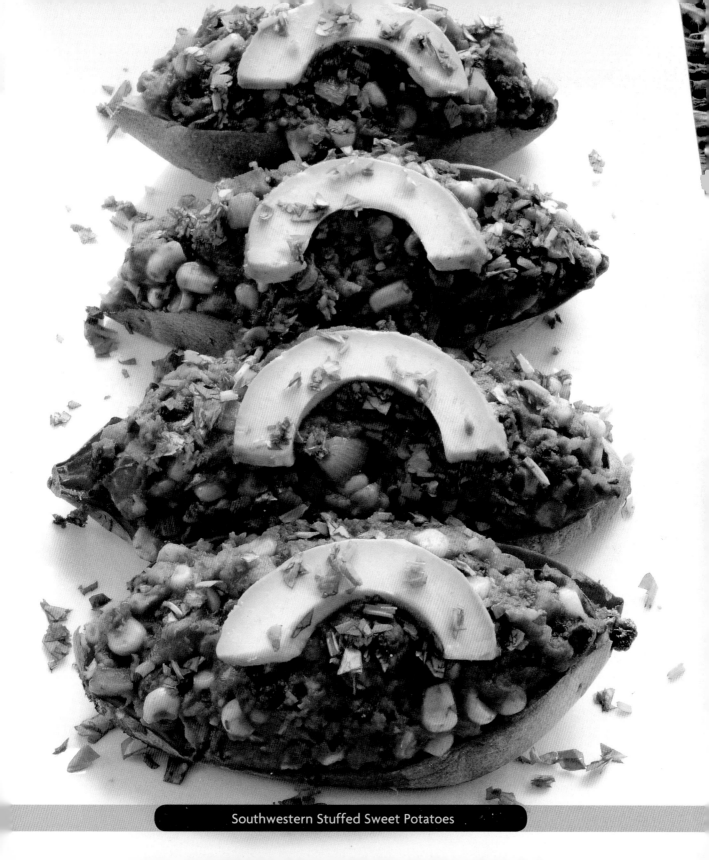

Southwestern Stuffed Sweet Potatoes

While the sweet potatoes are baking, prepare the filling. Put the onion, bell pepper, water, and garlic in a medium saucepan and cook over medium heat, stirring once or twice, until the vegetables are tender, about 5 minutes. Add the beans, corn, tomatoes, cumin, chili powder, and smoked paprika and stir to combine. Decrease the heat to medium-low and cook, stirring occasionally, for 15 minutes.

Cut the sweet potatoes in half lengthwise. Scoop out the flesh with a spoon, leaving enough so the skin remains firm and holds its shape. Put the sweet potato shells back in the oven to keep warm. Add the flesh to the filling mixture in the saucepan and stir until well distributed. Cook, stirring occasionally, for 10 minutes. Remove from the heat and stir in the cilantro and lime juice. Add the optional salt and season with pepper and optional hot sauce to taste. Spoon the filling into the sweet potato shells. Garnish with the avocado. Top with dollops of Cashew Mayonnaise if desired.

Tacos in a Bowl

MAKES 3 SERVINGS

The well-loved taco is an almost-instant meal, yet it's surprisingly nutritionally balanced. Since the filling is everyone's favorite part, these tacos are served in bowls instead of in taco shells. Simply warm the beans, chop the veggies, and set out the colorful fillings in pretty bowls.

1½ cups (375 ml) **cooked or canned black beans or pinto beans, mashed**

2 cups (500 ml) **shredded or chopped romaine or other lettuce**

1 cup (250 ml) **diced tomatoes**

1 cup (250 ml) **salsa**

1 **carrot, grated**

1 **avocado, diced**

Put the beans in a small saucepan and warm over medium-low heat. If they're too thick or stick to the pan, add a small amount of water. Alternatively, warm the beans in the microwave. Put the beans, lettuce, tomatoes, salsa, carrot, and avocado in separate bowls on the table so everyone can create their favorite combination.

VARIATIONS: Replace the avocado with Limey Avocado Dip, page 105. Replace the beans with vegan ground round.

Per serving:
calories: 276
protein: 10 g
fat: 11 g
carbohydrate: 38 g
dietary fiber: 16 g
calcium: 56 mg
sodium: 496 mg

Nori Rolls with Cauliflower Rice

MAKES 3 ROLLS,
7 PIECES PER ROLL

Plant-based nori rolls are delicious and fun to make. Using cauliflower instead of rice keeps the starch and calories low. Serve these rolls with wasabi paste and tamari for dipping.

2½ cups (625 ml) **cauliflower florets**

½ teaspoon (2 ml) **salt**

1 tablespoon (15 ml) **nutritional yeast flakes**

1 tablespoon (15 ml) **Date Paste (page 172)**

1 tablespoon (15 ml) **rice vinegar**

½ teaspoon (2 ml) **ground turmeric**

6 sheets **nori**

¼ **red or orange bell pepper, cut into long, thin strips**

¼ **cucumber, peeled and cut into long, thin strips the length of the cucumber**

1 **green onion, cut into long, thin strips**

1 **avocado, cut in half, then cut into strips the length of the avocado**

1 cup (250 ml) **alfalfa sprouts**

½ cup (125 ml) **fresh herbs, such as basil, cilantro, dill, or parsley, lightly packed**

Put the cauliflower in a food processor and pulse into the texture of rice. If there are any large chunks remaining, mash them with a spoon. Transfer to a small bowl and sprinkle with the salt. Mix well and let sit for at least 20 minutes. Transfer to a fine-mesh sieve and squeeze the cauliflower with your hands to remove as much liquid as possible. Put the cauliflower back in the bowl. Add the nutritional yeast, Date Paste, vinegar, and turmeric and stir until well combined.

To assemble the rolls, put two nori sheets on a sushi mat (see Tip). Sprinkle about ½ cup (125 ml) of the cauliflower mixture over the nori and press it into a rectangle, leaving a wide margin on all sides. Lay the bell pepper, cucumber, green onion, avocado, sprouts, and herbs over the length of the cauliflower mixture. Gently bring the nori sheets up and over the filling and gently but

Per roll:
calories: 150
protein: 5 g
fat: 10 g
carbohydrate: 14 g
dietary fiber: 8 g
calcium: 53 mg
sodium: 425 mg

firmly roll up the nori sheets to create a log. Dip your finger in water and run it along the edge of one side of the nori, then fold over the other edge and press gently to seal the log. Gently roll the log back and forth to shape it before carefully cutting it with a sharp knife into six or eight pieces. Put the rolls on a serving platter, cut-side up. The ends of the rolls will have filling sticking out and will add a decorative flair. Repeat with the remaining nori sheets and filling to make three rolls (eighteen or twenty-four pieces) in all.

Put a sheet of plastic wrap over the sushi mat to prevent the nori from sticking to the mat.

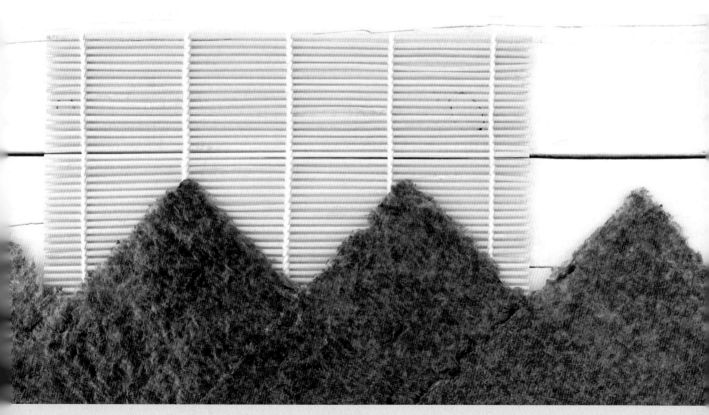

Beet and Lentil Patties

MAKES 8 PATTIES

Crunchy on the outside, chewy on the inside, these baked burgers can be eaten between romaine lettuce leaves or on a plate with a side of salad. They store well in the fridge or freezer.

½ cup (125 ml) **old-fashioned rolled oats**

½ cup (125 ml) **sunflower seeds or walnuts**

2 cups (500 ml) **grated beets**

¼ cup (60 ml) **ground flaxseeds**

2 teaspoons (10 ml) **dried thyme**

1 teaspoon (5 ml) **ground fennel seeds**

1 onion, **coarsely chopped**

1 cup (250 ml) **coarsely chopped mushrooms**

¼ cup (60 ml) **coarsely chopped garlic**

¼ cup (60 ml) **water**

2 cups (500 ml) **cooked or canned brown lentils, drained and rinsed**

1 cup (250 ml) **cooked quinoa or brown rice**

½ teaspoon (2 ml) **salt**

Freshly ground black pepper

Put the oats and sunflower seeds in a food processor and pulse into a coarse meal. Transfer to a large bowl. Add the beets, flaxseeds, thyme, and fennel seeds and stir until well combined. Set aside.

Put the onion, mushrooms, garlic, and water in a medium skillet. Cover and cook over medium heat, stirring occasionally, until the vegetables are tender but not mushy, about 10 minutes. Let cool, then transfer to the food processor. Add the lentils and rice and pulse until well combined but still chunky, stopping occasionally to scrape down the work bowl. Add to the bowl with the oats and stir until well combined. Add the salt and season with pepper to taste.

Preheat the oven to 375 degrees F (190 degrees C). Line a baking sheet with parchment paper or a silicone baking mat.

Per patty:

calories: 217

protein: 11 g

fat: 7 g

carbohydrate: 31 g

dietary fiber: 10 g

calcium: 64 mg

sodium: 188 mg

Flatten the top of the lentil mixture in the bowl and use a knife to cut the mixture into eight equal wedges. Form each wedge into a ball, then flatten the balls into patties. Put the patties on the lined baking sheet as they are formed. Bake for 20 minutes, flip the patties over, and bake for 20 minutes longer, until brown and crispy.

HERBED BEET AND LENTIL PATTIES: Add 1 tablespoon (15 ml) tamari, 1 teaspoon (5 ml) dried oregano, 1 teaspoon (5 ml) dry mustard, 1 teaspoon (5 ml) dried thyme, 1 teaspoon (5 ml) dried sage, and ½ teaspoon (2 ml) salt.

SPICED BEET AND LENTIL PATTIES: Omit the fennel seeds and thyme and add 2 tablespoons (30 ml) tamari, 2 teaspoons (10 ml) apple cider vinegar, ½ teaspoon (2 ml) ground coriander, ½ teaspoon (2 ml) ground cumin, ½ teaspoon (2 ml) paprika, and ½ teaspoon (2 ml) ground turmeric.

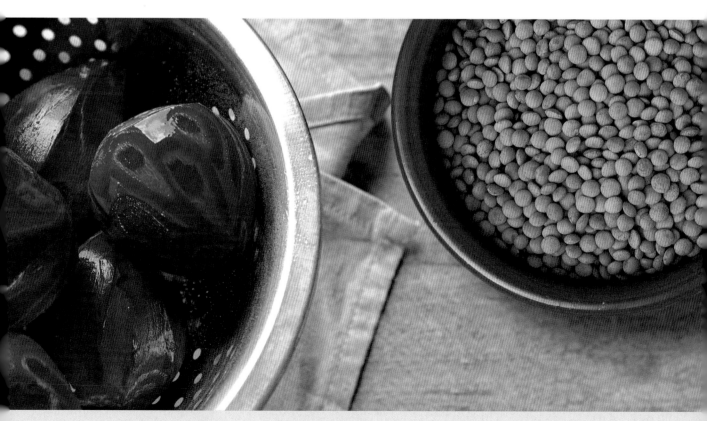

Black Beans and Greens

MAKES 6½ CUPS
(1.63 L),
4 SERVINGS

Beans and greens are the ultimate disease-fighting food combination. The wealth of herbs and spices in this dish further enhance its antioxidants and rich flavor. Serve it alongside a baked sweet potato or your favorite intact whole grain. Add a steamed vegetable or salad and dinner is done!

1¾ cups (435 ml) **water or vegetable broth**

2 cups (500 ml) **diced carrots**

1 medium onion, **chopped**

1 cup (250 ml) **chopped celery**

1 bell pepper (any color), **diced**

2½ cups (625 ml) **cooked or canned black beans, drained and rinsed**

1 teaspoon (5 ml) **paprika**

1 teaspoon (5 ml) **garlic powder**

1 teaspoon (5 ml) **dried oregano**

1 teaspoon (5 ml) **dried thyme**

½ teaspoon (2 ml) **ground black pepper**

½ teaspoon (2 ml) **cayenne** (optional)

¼ teaspoon (1 ml) **salt**

3 cups (750 ml) **stemmed and thinly sliced dark leafy greens** (such as collard greens, kale, spinach, or Swiss chard), **packed**

2 green onions, **thinly sliced**

Put ¼ cup (60 ml) of the water and the carrots, onion, celery, and bell pepper in a large saucepan. Cook over medium heat, stirring occasionally, until the vegetables are tender, about 10 minutes. Add the remaining 1½ cups (375 ml) of the water and the beans, paprika, garlic powder, oregano, thyme, pepper, optional cayenne, and salt. Bring to a boil over medium-high heat. Add the greens, decrease the heat to medium-low, cover, and cook until the greens are tender, 5–10 minutes. Stir, remove from the heat, cover, and let sit for 10 minutes to allow the flavors to blend. Sprinkle with the green onions just before serving.

Per serving
(1⅝ cups/415 ml):
calories: 222
protein: 13 g
fat: 1 g
carbohydrate: 44 g
dietary fiber: 14 g
calcium: 152 mg
sodium: 232 mg

Note: Analysis done with Swiss chard.

10

SWEET
TREATS

Apple Crisp

MAKES 9 SERVINGS

nce the chopping is done, this dessert pulls together in just a few minutes. Crunchy and naturally sweet, it will satisfy your cravings for a treat. If you like, top each serving with a dollop of Cashew-Pear Cream (page 171).

5 cups (1.25 L) thinly sliced apples

2 tablespoons (30 ml) finely chopped dates

2 tablespoons (30 ml) lemon juice

1 teaspoon (5 ml) ground cinnamon

¼ cup (60 ml) water

2 tablespoons (30 ml) Date Paste (page 172)

2 tablespoons (30 ml) almond butter

1 teaspoon (5 ml) vanilla extract

1½ cups (375 ml) old-fashioned rolled oats

¼ cup (60 ml) chopped walnuts

¼ cup (60 ml) sunflower seeds

Preheat the oven to 350 degrees F (175 degrees C).

Put the apples, dates, lemon juice, and cinnamon in an 8-inch (20-cm) square baking dish. Stir to combine, then press down the apples to flatten them evenly into the pan.

Put the water, Date Paste, almond butter, and vanilla extract in a medium bowl and stir until well combined. Add the oats, walnuts, and sunflower seeds and stir until very well combined, scraping the bowl occasionally to incorporate any mixture that sticks on the bottom. Layer evenly over the apples and press down with the back of a spoon, metal spatula, or moistened hands to flatten and pack down the mixture. Bake for 25–35 minutes, until the apples are very soft.

Per serving:

calories: 168

protein: 4 g

fat: 7 g

carbohydrate: 25 g

dietary fiber: 5 g

calcium: 33 mg

sodium: 17 mg

Fresh Fruit Salad

MAKES 5 CUPS
(1.25 L)

Fruit is an appealing accompaniment to breakfast, a welcome snack to boost energy in the afternoon, and a sweet way to end the day. This salad combines the tang of grapefruit, the crunch of apple, the sweetness of banana, the zing of orange, and the protective power of berries.

1 grapefruit, separated into segments

1 apple or pear, diced

1 banana, sliced

1 cup (250 ml) berries (any kind) or sliced strawberries

Juice of 1 orange

1 sprig fresh mint, chopped (optional)

Put the grapefruit, apple, banana, and berries in a medium bowl. Add the orange juice and stir gently to combine. Garnish with the optional mint.

Vary this salad with seasonal fruits or berries from the freezer. Treat yourself to organic whenever possible.

Per 1 cup (250 ml):

calories: 76

protein: 1 g

fat: 0.3 g

carbohydrate: 19 g

dietary fiber: 3 g

calcium: 9 mg

sodium: 1 mg

Stewed Fruit

MAKES 2½ CUPS
(625 ML)

Stewed fruit is a delightful addition to hot cereal or a Sweet Break-fast Bowl (page 59). It also makes a simple but delicious dessert, especially when topped with a little Cashew-Pear Cream (page 171), cinnamon, and Wholly Granola (page 60) or chopped walnuts.

4 cups (1 L) **fresh or frozen fruit** (such as apricots, berries, Italian prune plums, peaches, or nectarines, or a combination)

3 tablespoons (45 ml) **water**

Quarter the apricots and plums and dice or cube larger stone fruits. Put the fruit and water in a medium saucepan. Cover and cook over low heat, stirring occasionally, until the fruit it is soft, 30–45 minutes. Let cool. Stored in a sealed container in the refrigerator, Stewed Fruit will keep for 5 days.

Freeze fresh fruit when it's in season so you can make stewed fruit all year long.

Per 1¼ cups (310 ml):
calories: 118
protein: 3 g
fat: 0.8 g
carbohydrate: 28 g
dietary fiber: 6 g
calcium: 0 mg
sodium: 0 mg

Note: Analysis done with mixed berries.

Tutti Frutti Ice Cream

MAKES 4 SERVINGS

This simple nondairy dessert will remind you of soft-serve ice cream. It's high in potassium and protective phytochemicals and is sweet without added sugar.

2 large or 3 small bananas, peeled and frozen solid

2 cups (500 ml) frozen berries, cherries, diced mango, or pineapple chunks

⅓ cup (85 ml) fortified unsweetened soy milk or other nondairy milk

Put all the ingredients in a food processor and process until smooth. Serve immediately.

CHOCOLATE OR CAROB ICE CREAM: Add 1 tablespoon (15 ml) unsweetened cocoa or carob powder.

VANILLA ICE CREAM: Double the bananas and omit the other fruit. Add ½ teaspoon (2 ml) vanilla extract. Top with Very Berry Sauce (page 170) and chopped nuts if desired. If you like, include a few raisins or pitted dates for additional sweetness.

To process in a high-powered blender, increase the milk to ½ cup (125 ml). Begin processing on low and gradually increase the speed, pushing the fruit down with the tamper, until smooth.

Per serving:
calories: 91
protein: 2 g
fat: 1 g
carbohydrate: 22 g
dietary fiber: 3 g
calcium: 45 mg
sodium: 9 mg

Vanilla Chia Pudding

**MAKES 2 CUPS
(500 ML), 4 SERVINGS**

For a thicker pudding,
use ⅓ cup (85 ml) chia
seeds.

hia seed pudding makes a wonderful dessert or wholesome breakfast. If you like, top it with fresh berries or sliced fruit.

2 cups (500 ml) **fortified unsweetened soy milk or other nondairy milk**

¼ cup (60 ml) **pitted soft dates**

1 teaspoon (5 ml) **vanilla extract**

¼ cup (60 ml) **chia seeds**

Put the milk, dates, and vanilla extract in a blender and process until smooth.
Add the chia seeds and pulse until the seeds are distributed through the
liquid but not blended. Transfer to a storage container, cover tightly, and
refrigerate for at least 2 hours. Stir well before serving to break up any clumps
of chia seeds.

CHOCOLATE CHIA PUDDING: Add ¼ cup (60 ml) unsweetened cocoa or cacao
powder before processing.

Per serving
(½ cup/125 ml):
calories: 146
protein: 5 g
fat: 6 g
carbohydrate: 19 g
dietary fiber: 7 g
calcium: 271 mg
sodium: 50 mg

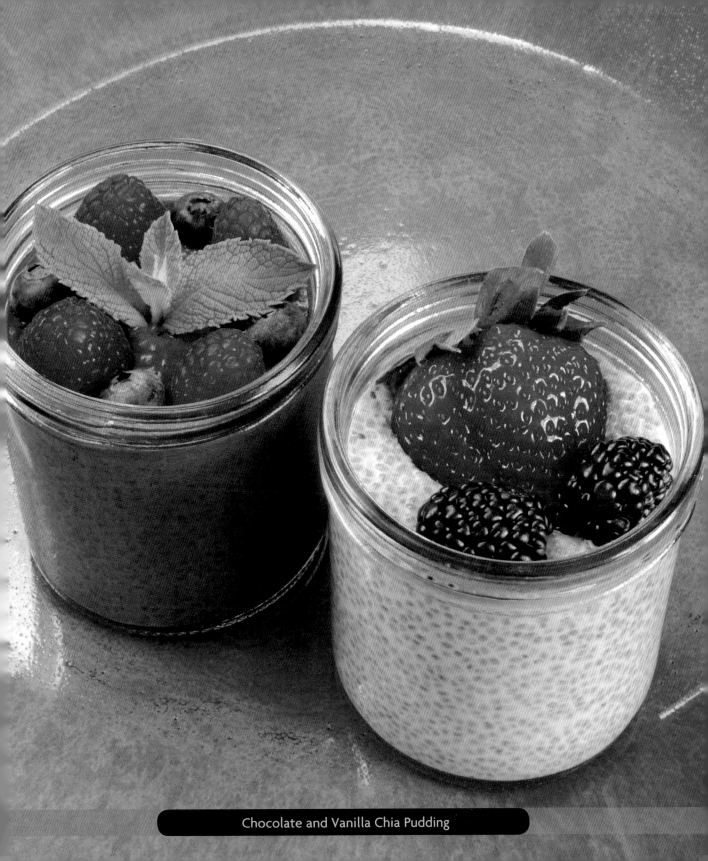

Chocolate and Vanilla Chia Pudding

Chewy Walnut Cookies

MAKES 26 COOKIES

These yummy cookies are rich in essential omega-3 fatty acids and are free of concentrated sweeteners, oil, and flour. If you like, decorate each cookie with a pecan or walnut half before baking.

1 cup (250 ml) pitted soft dates, firmly packed

½ cup (125 ml) water

3 tablespoons (45 ml) tahini

1 teaspoon (5 ml) vanilla extract

1 cup (250 ml) walnuts, very finely chopped

½ cup (125 ml) ground flaxseeds

½ cup (125 ml) unsweetened shredded dried coconut

¼ cup (60 ml) sesame seeds, sunflower seeds, or chia seeds

1 teaspoon (5 ml) ground cinnamon

¼ teaspoon (1 ml) salt (optional)

Preheat the oven to 350 degrees F (175 degrees C). Line two baking sheets with parchment paper or silicone baking mats.

Put the dates and water in a small saucepan and cook over medium heat, stirring occasionally, until the dates are very soft, about 5 minutes. Transfer to a medium bowl and mash with a potato masher. Add the tahini and vanilla extract and stir until well combined. Add the walnuts, flaxseeds, coconut, sesame seeds, cinnamon, and optional salt and stir until well combined.

Form into twenty-six equal balls, using about 2 tablespoons (30 ml) per ball. Arrange on the lined baking sheets and press down with a fork to flatten. If necessary, dip the fork in water to keep it from sticking. Bake for 12–15 minutes, or until lightly browned.

Per cookie:
calories: 85
protein: 3 g
fat: 6 g
carbohydrate: 7 g
dietary fiber: 2 g
calcium: 28 mg
sodium: 3 mg

Lime Bliss Balls

MAKES 30 BALLS

Rich, sweet, tangy, and tart, these little no-bake balls are a true delight. They'll satisfy the most insistent sweet tooth in need of a snack.

1 cup (250 ml) raw almonds

1 cup (250 ml) raw cashews

⅛ teaspoon (0.5 ml) salt

1 cup (250 ml) pitted soft dates

Zest and juice of 2 limes

1 cup (250 ml) unsweetened shredded dried coconut

¾ cup (185 ml) dried currants or other unsweetened dried fruit
   (such as cherries or finely chopped apricots, nectarines, or peaches)

Put the almonds, cashews, and salt in a food processor and process into a coarse flour. Transfer to a large bowl. Put the dates, lime zest, lime juice, and coconut in the food processor and process into a soft paste, stopping occasionally to scrape down the work bowl. Add the date paste to the nut flour. Add the currants and stir until well combined.

   Form the mixture into thirty equal balls, using about 2 tablespoons (30 ml) per ball. Roll the balls between your hands, pressing them firmly so they hold together. Arrange in a single layer in a flat storage container. Cover tightly and store in the refrigerator or freezer.

COATED BLISS BALLS: Roll the balls in unsweetened shredded dried coconut, slivered almonds, hemp seeds, lime zest, or sesame seeds.

PINK POMEGRANATE BLISS BALLS: Replace the lime juice with ¼ cup (60 ml) pomegranate juice and replace the almonds with hemp seeds.

Per ball:
calories 95
protein: 2 g
fat: 6 g
carbohydrate: 10 g
dietary fiber: 2 g
calcium: 22 mg
sodium: 11 mg

Black Bean Brownies

MAKES 16 BROWNIES

Top these healthy brownies with Chocolate Fudge Frosting (page 170), Cashew-Pear Cream (page 171) and berries, or Tutti Frutti Ice Cream (page 161). They freeze beautifully.

1½ cups (375 ml) **cooked or canned black beans, drained and rinsed**

¾ cup (185 ml) **pitted soft dates, packed**

⅓ cup (85 ml) **unsweetened cocoa powder**

3 tablespoons (45 ml) **almond butter or other nut butter**

3 tablespoons (45 ml) **ground chia seeds or flaxseeds**

1 teaspoon (5 ml) **vanilla extract**

½ cup (125 ml) **coarsely chopped walnuts**

Preheat the oven to 200 degrees F (95 degrees C). Mist an 8-inch (20-cm) square baking pan with cooking spray or line it with parchment paper.

Put the beans, dates, cocoa powder, almond butter, chia seeds, and vanilla extract in a food processor and process until smooth. Add the walnuts and pulse just until evenly distributed. Pat the mixture evenly into the prepared baking pan. Cover and bake for 1½ hours. Cool completely before cutting into squares.

Per brownie:

calories: 106

protein: 4 g

fat: 5 g

carbohydrate: 13 g

dietary fiber: 4 g

calcium: 31 mg

sodium: 1 mg

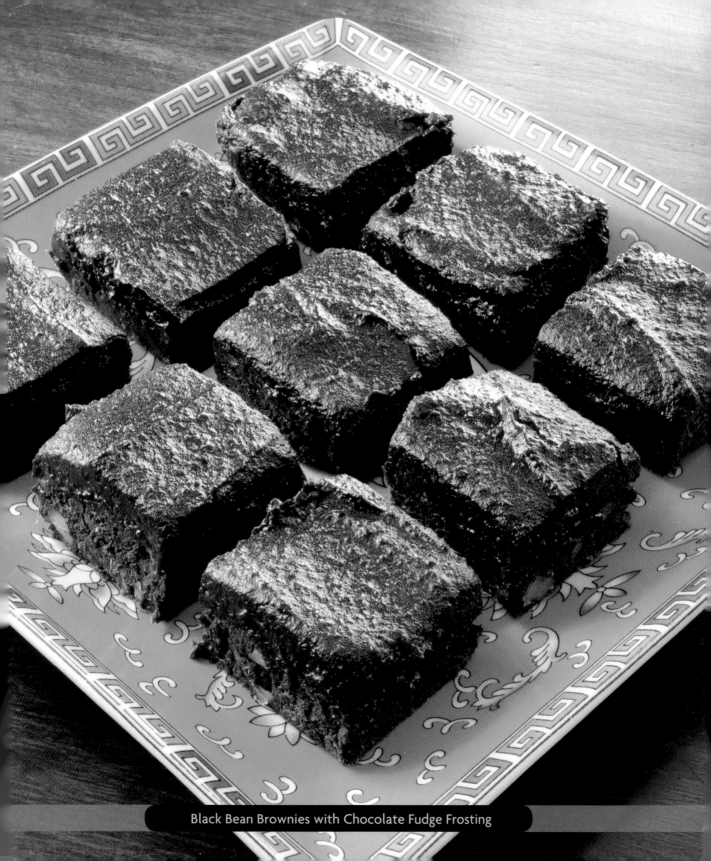

Black Bean Brownies with Chocolate Fudge Frosting

Stuffed Medjool Dates

**MAKES 24
STUFFED DATES**

Per 2 dates:

calories: 139

protein: 2 g

fat: 6 g

carbohydrate: 23 g

dietary fiber: 3 g

calcium: 37 mg

sodium: 24 mg

Save these elegant treats for a special occasion. They freeze beautifully. You can get creative with the decorations, but nuts work especially well.

24 large, soft medjool dates

1½ cups (375 ml) Chocolate Fudge Frosting (page 170)

72 roasted hazelnuts or almonds

Cut a slice in each date lengthwise, keeping the bottom of the dates and both ends intact, and remove the pit. Gently spread the dates open so there's room for the stuffing. Evenly stuff the dates with the frosting. Press the nuts on top of the frosting, using 3 nuts per date. Store the stuffed dates in a sealed container in the refrigerator or freezer.

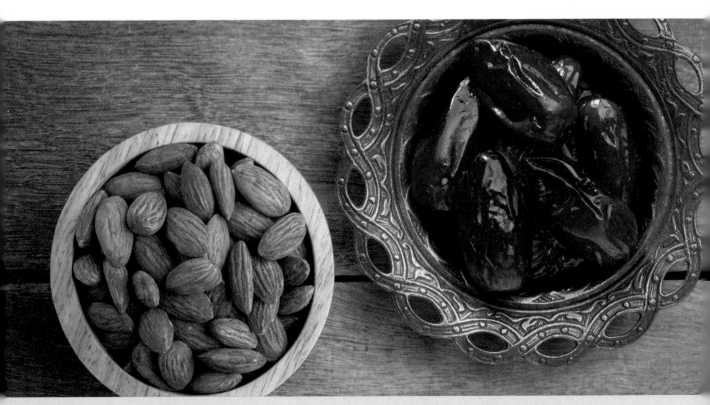

Pumpkin Parfaits

I f you love pumpkin pie, you'll be smitten with these parfaits. They capture all the irresistible flavors of the pie without the high-calorie crust, and they make a beautiful presentation.

MAKES 6 PARFAITS

3 cups (750 ml) **Cashew-Pear Cream** (page 171), chilled

1 can (15 ounces/425 g) **pumpkin puree** (see Tip)

½ cup (125 ml) **fortified unsweetened soy milk or other nondairy milk**

¼ cup (60 ml) **pitted soft dates, packed**

1 teaspoon (5 ml) **ground cinnamon, plus more for garnish**

½ teaspoon (2 ml) **ground ginger**

¼ teaspoon (1 ml) **ground cloves**

¼ teaspoon (1 ml) **ground nutmeg, plus more for garnish**

¾ cup (185 ml) **Wholly Granola** (page 60), chopped walnuts or pecans, or a combination of Wholly Granola and nuts

Put 1 cup (250 ml) of the Cashew-Pear Cream and the pumpkin, milk, dates, cinnamon, ginger, cloves, and nutmeg in a food processor and process until smooth.

Have ready six parfait glasses or tall glasses with stems. To assemble the parfaits, spoon 3 tablespoons (45 ml) of the pumpkin mixture into each glass. Top with about 2 tablespoons (30 ml) of the Cashew-Pear Cream and 2 teaspoons (10 ml) of the granola. Repeat the layers two more times. Garnish with a sprinkling of cinnamon and/or nutmeg if desired. Refrigerate for at least 2 hours before serving. Serve cold.

Be sure to use only pure pumpkin puree, not pumpkin pie filling. To boost the flavor even more, increase the seasonings to suit your taste, or use grated fresh ginger and nutmeg.

Per parfait:
calories: 233
protein: 5 g
fat: 9 g
carbohydrate: 38 g
dietary fiber: 5 g
calcium: 67 mg
sodium: 23 mg

Chocolate Fudge Frosting

MAKES 1½ CUPS
(375 ML)

Per 1 tablespoon (15 ml):
calories: 46
protein: 1 g
fat: 3 g
carbohydrate: 4 g
dietary fiber: 1 g
calcium: 17 mg
sodium: 24 mg

Note: Analysis was done using almond butter.

This makes enough to frost one batch of Black Bean Brownies (page 166) and also fill twelve Stuffed Medjool Dates (page 168). Alternatively, use it to fill twenty-four Stuffed Medjool Dates.

½ cup (125 ml) pitted soft dates, packed

½ cup (125 ml) boiling water

½ cup (125 ml) nut or seed butter

¼ cup (60 ml) unsweetened cocoa powder

1 teaspoon (5 ml) vanilla extract

Put the dates in a heatproof bowl. Add the boiling water and let soak until soft, about 10 minutes. Transfer the dates and the soaking liquid to a food processor. Add the nut butter, cocoa powder, and vanilla extract and process until smooth, stopping occasionally to scrape down the work bowl. Use immediately or store in a sealed container in the refrigerator. Bring to room temperature before using.

Very Berry Sauce

MAKES 2 CUPS (500 ML)

Per ¼ cup (60 ml):
calories: 22
protein: 0 g
fat: 0.1 g
carbohydrate: 5 g
dietary fiber: 1 g
calcium: 0 mg
sodium: 0 mg

Pour this scrumptious sauce over Banana-Walnut Pancakes (page 66) or Tutti Frutti Ice Cream (page 161).

2 cups (500 ml) fresh or frozen blueberries or raspberries

¼ cup (60 ml) water

2 teaspoons (10 ml) cornstarch or arrowroot starch mixed with 2 tablespoons (30 ml) water

Put the berries and water in a small saucepan and cook over medium heat, stirring occasionally, for 10 minutes. Stir the cornstarch mixture, then stir it into the simmering berries. Cook, stirring constantly, until the sauce thickens, about 1 minute. Serve warm or cold.

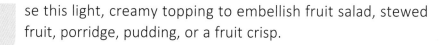

Cashew-Pear Cream

Use this light, creamy topping to embellish fruit salad, stewed fruit, porridge, pudding, or a fruit crisp.

MAKES 1¾ CUPS
(435 ML)

1 can (14 ounces/398 ml) **pears packed in water or juice**

½ cup (125 ml) **raw cashews**

½ teaspoon (2 ml) **vanilla extract**

Drain the pears but reserve the liquid. Put the pears, cashews, and vanilla extract in a blender and process until smooth, 1–2 minutes. Add some of the liquid from the pears to achieve the desired consistency. Stored in a sealed container in the refrigerator, the cream will keep for 4 days.

Per ¼ cup (60 ml):
calories: 88
protein: 2 g
fat: 4 g
carbohydrate: 12 g
dietary fiber: 1 g
calcium: 3 mg
sodium: 6 mg

Date Paste

MAKES 1 CUP
(250 ML)

Date paste is the ideal substitute for refined sugar. While most sweeteners have no fiber and few nutrients, date paste is made from only dates and water, so it provides all the fiber and nutrients found in the whole food. It can be used to sweeten puddings, sauces, salad dressings, baked goods, and raw treats. Recent research suggests that dates have a low glycemic index of 43–55, depending on the variety. This adds to their appeal as a sweetener, but they should still be used in very small amounts.

> 1 cup (250 ml) pitted soft dates, packed, coarsely chopped
> ⅔ cup (165 ml) boiling water

Put the dates and water in a blender and process until smooth, stopping occasionally to scrape down the blender jar. Stored in a sealed container in the refrigerator, the paste will keep for 3 weeks.

If the dates are hard or dry, steam them or soak them in the boiling water for 15–30 minutes before blending or processing. A food processor also works well for this recipe, so if your blender isn't very powerful, use a food processor instead. Use the smaller processor bowl, if you have one, or a mini processor.

Per 1 tablespoon (15 ml):
calories: 31
protein: 0 g
fat: 0 g
carbohydrate: 8 g
dietary fiber: 1 g
calcium: 4 mg
sodium: 0 mg

INDEX

Recipe titles appear in *italics*.

A

African Chickpea Stew, 132
alcohol consumption, 8, 17, 18
animal products and/or meat
    calories from fat and, 11
    fiber in, lack of, 1
    as food foe/unhealthy, 2, 9, 11,
       17, 22
    minimizing consumption of, 8
    veggie meats as substitute for,
       29, 32
antioxidants
    in fruits, 29
    in herbs and/or spices, 39
    in legumes, 9
    in nuts and/or seeds, 36, 37, 38
    in plant foods, 2, 7, 13, 14
    Recommended Dietary
       Allowance (RDA) for, 15
    in starchy vegetables, 33
    in whole grains, 34
apple(s)
    Crisp, 158
    Red Cabbage and, 122
    -Spice Oatmeal, Baked, 63
arsenic in foods, 14, 56
artificial sweeteners, 7, 8, 21
Asian Green Beans, 124
avocado(s)
    *Avocado, Kamut, Kale, and
       Tomato Salad,* 100
    Dip or Dressing, Limey, 105

    in *Green Potato Salad with Dill,*
       87
    and *Kale Soup,* 74

B

bad bacteria (dysbiosis), 7, 8
baked dishes/recipes
    Apple-Spice Oatmeal, 63
    *Potatoes or Sweet Potatoes,
       Full-Meal,* 139
    Squash Casserole, 127
baking foods, 27
Balls, Lime Bliss (and variations),
    165
Banana-Walnut Pancakes, 66
barley
    *Barley, Split Pea, and Lentil
       Soup, Hearty,* 77
    *Barley, Sun-Dried Tomato, and
       Bean Salad,* 99
    and *Beans Soup, Full of,* 81
    and *Oat Groat Porridge,* 62
Base, Better Broth, 71
basil, in *Walnut Pesto,* 111
Basmati Rice and Cauliflower Salad,
    94
bean(s). *See also* specific types of
    and *Barley Soup, Full of,* 81
    *Bean, Barley, and Sun-Dried
       Tomato Salad,* 99
    *Beans, Greens, and Sweet
       Potato with Tahini-Lime
       Sauce,* 64
    in Native American dish, 136

Becoming Vegan (express/
    comprehensive editions), 16
beet(s)
    Hummus, Blushing, 113
    and *Lentil Patties* (and
       variations), 154–155
    in *Ruby Red Salad,* 93
berry(ies)
    contaminants and, 14
    as food friend, 17, 28
    in fruit water, 29
    Sauce, Very, 170–171
Better Broth Base, 71
The Big Easy Bowl, 131
bisphenol A (BPA), 15, 27, 32
black bean(s)
    Brownies, 166
    Chili, Sweet Potato and, 133
    and *Greens,* 155
    Hummus, 113
    and *Mango Salad,* 98
    Soup, Zesty, 76
Black-Eyed Pea and Eggplant Soup,
    83
blanching foods, 27
Blend Soup, Garden, 73
Bliss Balls, Lime (and variations), 165
blood sugar
    artificial sweeteners and, 7
    bread and, 36
    caffeine and, 18
    cinnamon and, 4, 38, 39
    citrus fruits and, 28
    dried fruits and, 29

TABLE A.1 Dietary reference intakes for vitamins

AGE / LIFE STAGE	VIT A mcg	VIT C mg	VIT D mcg	VIT E mg	VIT K mcg	THIAMIN mg	RIBOFLAVIN mg	NIACIN mg	VIT B_6 mg	FOLATE mcg	VIT B_{12} mcg	PANTOTHENIC ACID mg	BIOTIN mcg	CHOLINE mg
INFANTS														
0–6 months	400	40	10	4	2.0	0.2	0.3	2	0.1	65	0.4	1.7	5	125
7–12 months	500	50	10	5	2.5	0.3	0.4	4	0.3	80	0.5	1.8	6	150
CHILDREN														
1–3 years	300	15	15	6	30	0.5	0.5	6	0.5	150	0.9	2	8	200
4–8 years	400	25	15	7	55	0.6	0.6	8	0.6	200	1.2	3	12	250
MALES														
9–13 years	600	45	15	11	60	0.9	0.9	12	1.0	300	1.8	4	20	375
14–18 years	900	75	15	15	75	1.2	1.3	16	1.3	400	2.4	5	25	550
19–30 years	900	90	15	15	120	1.2	1.3	16	1.3	400	2.4	5	30	550
31–50 years	900	90	15	15	120	1.2	1.3	16	1.3	400	2.4	5	30	550
51–70 years	900	90	15	15	120	1.2	1.3	16	1.7	400	2.4	5	30	550
> 70 years	900	90	20	15	120	1.2	1.3	16	1.7	400	2.4	5	30	550
FEMALES														
9–13 years	600	45	15	11	60	0.9	0.9	12	1.0	300	1.8	4	20	375
14–18 years	700	65	15	15	75	1.0	1.0	14	1.2	400	2.4	5	25	400
19–30 years	700	75	15	15	90	1.1	1.1	14	1.3	400	2.4	5	30	425
31–50 years	700	75	15	15	90	1.1	1.1	14	1.3	400	2.4	5	30	425
51–70 years	700	75	15	15	90	1.1	1.1	14	1.5	400	2.4	5	30	425
> 70 years	700	75	20	15	90	1.1	1.1	14	1.5	400	2.4	5	30	425
PREGNANCY														
14–18 years	750	80	15	15	75	1.4	1.4	18	1.9	600	2.6	6	30	450
19–30 years	770	85	15	15	90	1.4	1.4	18	1.9	600	2.6	6	30	450
31–50 years	770	85	15	15	90	1.4	1.4	18	1.9	600	2.6	6	30	450
LACTATION														
14–18 years	1,200	115	15	19	75	1.4	1.6	17	2	500	2.8	7	35	550
19–30 years	1,300	120	15	19	90	1.4	1.6	17	2	500	2.8	7	35	550
31–50 years	1,300	120	15	19	90	1.4	1.6	17	2	500	2.8	7	35	550

Key: mcg = microgram, mg = milligram, g = gram

TABLE A.2 Dietary reference intakes for minerals

LIFE STAGE / AGE	CALCIUM mg	CHROMIUM mcg	COPPER mcg	FLUORIDE mg	IODINE mcg	IRON mg	MAGNESIUM mg	MANGANESE mg	MOLYBDENUM mcg	PHOSPHORUS mg	SELENIUM mcg	ZINC mg	POTASSIUM g	SODIUM g	CHLORIDE g
INFANTS															
0–6 months	200	0.2	200	0.01	110	0.27	30	0.003	2	100	15	2	0.4	0.12	0.18
7–12 months	260	5.5	220	0.5	130	11	75	0.6	3	275	20	3	0.7	0.37	0.57
CHILDREN															
1–3 years	700	11	340	0.7	90	7	80	1.2	17	460	20	3	3.0	1.0	1.5
4–8 years	1,000	15	440	1	90	10	130	1.5	22	500	30	5	3.8	1.2	1.9
MALES															
9–13 years	1,300	25	700	2	120	8	240	1.9	34	1,250	40	8	4.5	1.5	2.3
14–18 years	1,300	35	890	3	150	11	410	2.2	43	1,250	55	11	4.7	1.5	2.3
19–30 years	1,000	35	900	4	150	8	400	2.3	45	700	55	11	4.7	1.5	2.3
31–50 years	1,000	35	900	4	150	8	420	2.3	45	700	55	11	4.7	1.5	2.3
51–70 years	1,000	30	900	4	150	8	420	2.3	45	700	55	11	4.7	1.3	2.0
> 70 years	1,200	30	900	4	150	8	420	2.3	45	700	55	11	4.7	1.2	1.8
FEMALES															
9–13 years	1,300	21	700	2	120	8	240	1.6	34	1,250	40	8	4.5	1.5	2.3
14–18 years	1,300	24	890	3	150	15	360	1.6	43	1,250	55	9	4.7	1.5	2.3
19–30 years	1,000	25	900	3	150	18	310	1.8	45	700	55	8	4.7	1.5	2.3
31–50 years	1,000	25	900	3	150	18	320	1.8	45	700	55	8	4.7	1.5	2.3
51–70 years	1,200	20	900	3	150	8	320	1.8	45	700	55	8	4.7	1.3	2.0
> 70 years	1,200	20	900	3	150	8	320	1.8	45	700	55	8	4.7	1.2	1.8
PREGNANCY															
14–18 years	1,300	29	1,000	3	220	27	400	2.0	50	1,250	60	13	4.7	1.5	2.3
19–30 years	1,000	30	1,000	3	220	27	350	2.0	50	700	60	11	4.7	1.5	2.3
31–50 years	1,000	30	1,000	3	220	27	360	2.0	50	700	60	11	4.7	1.5	2.3
LACTATION															
14–18 years	1,300	44	1,300	3	290	10	360	2.6	50	1,250	70	14	5.1	1.5	2.3
19–30 years	1,000	45	1,300	3	290	9	310	2.6	50	700	70	12	5.1	1.5	2.3
31–50 years	1,000	45	1,300	3	290	9	320	2.6	50	700	70	12	5.1	1.5	2.3

Key mcg = microgram, mg = milligram, g = gram

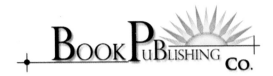

BOOK PUBLISHING CO.

books that educate, inspire, and empower

To find your favorite books on plant-based cooking and nutrition,
raw-foods cuisine, and healthy living, visit:
BookPubCo.com

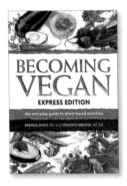

**Becoming Vegan
Express Edition**
*Brenda Davis, RD
Vesanto Melina, MS, RD*
978-1-57067-295-8 • $19.95

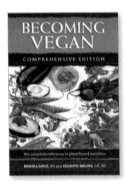

**Becoming Vegan
Comprehensive Edition**
*Brenda Davis, RD
Vesanto Melina, MS, RD*
978-1-57067-297-2 • $29.95

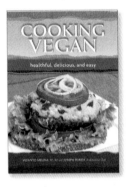

Cooking Vegan
*Vesanto Melina, MS, RD
Joseph Forest*
978-1-57067-267-5 • $19.95

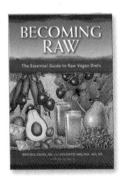

Becoming Raw
*Brenda Davis, RD
Vesanto Melina, MS, RD*
978-1-57067-238-5 • $24.95

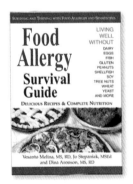

**Food Allergy
Survival Guide**
*Vesanto Melina, MS, RD
Jo Stepaniak, MSEd
Dina Aronson, MS, RD*
978-1-57067-163-0 • $19.95

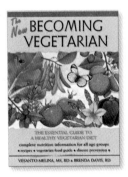

**The New
Becoming Vegetarian**
*Vesanto Melina, MS, RD
Brenda Davis, RD*
978-1-57067-144-9 • $21.95

Purchase these titles from your favorite book source or buy them directly from:
Book Publishing Company • PO Box 99 • Summertown, TN 38483 • 1-888-260-8458
Free shipping and handling on all orders